*Placement for Dementia*

# *Placement for Dementia*

A Dementia Care Essentials Guide

**PETER M. ABRAHAM, BSN, RN**

Placement for Dementia
A Dementia Care Essentials Guide
Copyright © 2024 Peter M. Abraham, BSN, RN

All rights reserved. No part of this book may be reproduced or transmitted in any manner whatsoever without written permission, except for brief quotations embodied in critical articles and reviews. This book is a work of nonfiction intended for educational purposes only.

This book is a work of non-fiction. The views expressed are solely those of the author and do not necessarily reflect the publisher's opinions, and the publisher hereby disclaims any responsibility for them.

Contact Info: author@2abraham.com

First Edition: August 2024

# DEDICATION

This book and the Dementia Care Essentials series it is part of are dedicated to multiple parties that helped shape my experiences and wisdom in caring for loved ones suffering from various types of dementia. I've worked with loved ones with dementia in long-term care as a registered nurse supervisor and as a hospice case manager. Caregivers and family members provided the most significant insights over the years.

Deborah, the wife of an Alzheimer's hospice at-home patient, provided insight into how the brains of dementia patients can be thought of like an electric clock. Most of the time, the clock is short-circuited and, therefore, not working correctly, but at times, as the clock's hands turn, the short-circuit goes away. For a fleeting time, a day or so, the person appears as if they don't have dementia.

Kathy is one of four daughters of a dementia patient for whom I provided care in a memory care center raised thought-provoking questions about the ethical dilemma of waking loved ones with dementia who want to sleep all the time to feed them vs. just letting them sleep.

Linda, who worked alongside me with a dementia patient, a former registered nurse herself, helped me understand other applications of validation therapy (a set of strategies and techniques that will be discussed in this book), such as rolling with resistance, which included accepting the nickname of "Jack," rather than my desire to be called Peter.

Jed, for whom I cared for his mother at home and then within a memory care center, reminded me of the actual cost that cannot be measured in terms of money of being a family caregiver.

Then there's our family journey, where my mother-in-law developed mixed dementia -- Alzheimer's disease plus vascular dementia – and was being cared for at home by her late husband, and then in a memory care center after he died suddenly.

More family members are involved, each helping me gain wisdom not taught in books. It is to all of these families and caregivers, as well as my late mother-in-law, Loris, and my wife, Laura, to whom this book and the others in this series are dedicated.

# Table of Contents

*Introduction* ............................................................. 1

*Caring for the Caregiver* ........................................ 2

   The Emotional and Physical Toll ........................ 2

   Recognizing the Signs of Caregiver Burnout ....... 3

   Understanding the Importance of Self-Care ........ 6

   Physical Self-Care Strategies ............................ 10

   Emotional and Mental Well-being ..................... 16

   Journaling and Emotional Expression ............... 18

   Seeking Professional Mental Health Support .... 20

   Utilizing Community Resources and Respite Care ....... 26

   Coping with Grief and Loss ............................. 40

   Finding Meaning in the Caregiving Journey ...... 42

   Self-Advocacy and Setting Boundaries ............. 44

   Continuing Education and Skills Development ... 46

*Planning: Legal and Financial Considerations* ....... 50

   Financial and Legal Considerations ................... 50

   Understanding Legal Rights and Options ......... 52

   Medical Power of Attorney: What It Is and Why It Matters ... 54

   Financial Power of Attorney: Protecting Assets and Finances ... 55

   Living Wills and Advance Directives ................. 56

   When and How to Have These Conversations .... 56

   Finding Legal Assistance for Document Preparation ... 57

   Exploring Financial Assistance Programs .......... 59

*Validation Therapy* ............................................. 62

   Naomi Feil's Validation Therapy ....................... 62

   Other Validation Techniques ........................... 65

   Environmental Modifications ........................... 68

   Practical Strategies for Caregivers ................... 69

    Communication Tips for De-escalating Fear ............... 71
    Case Studies and Real-Life Examples ..................... 73

*Navigating Placement* ............................................. *75*
    Recognizing When More Care Is Needed .................. 75
    Understanding Care Facility Options ....................... 78
    Financial Considerations for Long-Term Care ............ 81
    Choosing the Right Facility .................................. 85
    Navigating Facility Admissions ............................. 89
    Enhancing Home Care When Facility Placement Isn't an Option ............................................................. 93
    Making the Decision: Emotional and Practical Considerations _96

*Preparing for End-of-Life Decisions* ......................... *100*
*When to Consider Hospice* ..................................... *102*
    The importance of timely hospice involvement ......... 103
    Signs It May Be Time for Hospice Care .................. 104
    The Benefits of Hospice Care for Dementia Patients ... 107
    Respite care for family caregivers ......................... 108
    Improved quality of life ...................................... 109
    Common Misconceptions About Hospice Care ......... 110
    How to Initiate the Hospice Conversation .............. 114
    The Hospice Evaluation Process ........................... 117
    Preparing for Hospice Care .................................. 121
    Navigating the Emotional Journey ......................... 124
    Legal and Financial Considerations ....................... 128

*Conclusion* ............................................................ *132*
*Resources* ............................................................. *133*
*Author Bio* ............................................................ *134*

# Introduction

I know caring for someone with dementia can be challenging, especially when you are uncertain if your loved one can remain safe at home or you don't think they can move in with you. As an experienced nurse who's worked in long-term care and hospice, I've seen firsthand how difficult it can be for families and caregivers.

Taking care of a loved one with dementia is already a big task. They might not even realize they have dementia, which can make things even trickier. It's like they're moving forward in time physically, but mentally and emotionally, and functionally, they're heading back to being entirely dependent, kind of like a newborn.

That's why I wanted to write this book. I hope it'll give you some helpful strategies for making the decision as to when it's time to place your loved one in a facility. And if that's not possible, then what? And don't worry—many of these tips will also benefit other aspects of caregiving!

I've set up this book with you in mind. We'll start by discussing why it's so crucial for you to take care of yourself. When someone you love has a serious, long-term illness like dementia (which can last for decades), it affects the whole family. The person with dementia isn't the only one suffering - caregivers like you are going through a lot, too.

After we cover self-care and some practical tips, we will discuss the importance of early legal and financial planning, which is crucial to protect yourself and your loved one. Then, we'll discuss validation therapy and other ways to communicate better with your loved one. Trust me, these skills will come in handy in all sorts of tricky situations, not just with dementia care.

Once we've covered those basics, we'll get into the nitty-gritty of making a decision to place your loved one, including learning about the various types of facilities and their pros and cons. Since many people with dementia eventually need end-of-life care, we'll wrap up by covering that vital topic, too.

I'm here to help you through this journey. It isn't easy, but you can do it with the right tools and support. Remember, you're not alone in this!

# Caring for the Caregiver

Caring for a loved one with dementia is a journey of profound love and dedication, but it's also one of the most challenging roles a person can undertake. As caregivers and family members, you stand at the forefront of this complex and often overwhelming experience. Your commitment to providing compassionate care is admirable, yet it's crucial to recognize the significant impact this role can have on your well-being.

## The Emotional and Physical Toll

The path of a dementia caregiver is paved with a myriad of emotions and physical demands that can test even the strongest individuals. Let's explore the multifaceted nature of this toll:

**Emotional Challenges:**

1. Grief and loss: Watching a loved one's cognitive decline
2. Guilt: Feeling inadequate or struggling with difficult decisions
3. Anxiety: Worrying about the future and managing daily uncertainties
4. Frustration: Dealing with repetitive behaviors and communication barriers
5. Isolation: Experiencing a shrinking social circle and loss of personal time

**Physical Demands:**

- Sleep deprivation due to irregular sleep patterns of the care recipient
- Chronic stress leading to weakened immune function
- Neglect of personal health needs and medical appointments
- Physical strain from assisting with mobility and personal care tasks
- Exhaustion from constant vigilance and round-the-clock care

These emotional and physical challenges create a complex web that can entangle even the most resilient caregivers. It's essential to recognize that experiencing these difficulties doesn't reflect on your capabilities or dedication – it's a natural response to an extraordinarily demanding situation.

| Common Caregiver Emotions | Physical Manifestations | Potential Long-term Consequences |
|---|---|---|
| Sadness, Grief | Fatigue, Weakened Immunity | Depression, Chronic Illness |
| Anxiety, Worry | Insomnia, Muscle Tension | Anxiety Disorders, Chronic Pain |
| Frustration, Anger | High Blood Pressure, Headaches | Cardiovascular Issues, Migraines |
| Guilt, Self-doubt | Appetite Changes, Digestive Issues | Eating Disorders, Gastrointestinal Problems |

# Recognizing the Signs of Caregiver Burnout

Caregiver burnout is a state of physical, emotional, and mental exhaustion that can creep up slowly or suddenly. Awareness of the warning signs is crucial to prevent reaching this critical point. Here are key indicators to watch for:

1. **Emotional Signs:**
    - Feeling overwhelmed or constantly worried
    - Experiencing mood swings or irritability
    - Losing interest in activities once enjoyed
    - Feeling hopeless, helpless, or alone

2. **Physical Signs:**
    - Frequently falling ill or feeling constantly tired
    - Changes in appetite or sleep patterns
    - Neglecting personal hygiene or appearance
    - Developing new health problems or exacerbating existing ones

3. **Behavioral Signs:**
    - Withdrawing from friends and family
    - Procrastinating on important tasks
    - Using alcohol, food, or medications to cope
    - Lashing out at the person with dementia or others

4. **Cognitive Signs:**
    - Difficulty concentrating or making decisions
    - Forgetfulness in daily tasks
    - Trouble problem-solving or thinking clearly
    - Negative thought patterns or constant worry

## Self-Assessment Checklist for Caregiver Burnout:

| Warning Sign | Frequency (Rarely/Sometimes/Often/Always) |
| --- | --- |
| I feel exhausted even after sleeping. | |
| I catch myself yelling or arguing more often. | |
| I've stopped seeing friends or engaging in hobbies. | |
| I feel resentful towards the person I'm caring for. | |
| I worry constantly about the future. | |
| I neglect my own health needs. | |
| I have trouble falling asleep or staying asleep. | |
| I feel like I can't do anything right. | |

If you find yourself answering "Often" or "Always" to several of these statements, it may be time to seek additional support and focus on self-care strategies.

Remember, recognizing these signs is not an admission of failure but a crucial step in maintaining your ability to provide care. By acknowledging the challenges and being vigilant about your well-being, you can take proactive steps to prevent burnout and ensure that you can continue to provide the best possible care for your loved one with dementia. Your role is invaluable, and by taking care of yourself, you're also ensuring the best care for your loved one.

# Understanding the Importance of Self-Care

As caregivers and family members supporting individuals with dementia, you're intimately familiar with the concept of care. However, it's crucial to remember that care must also extend to you. Self-care isn't a luxury; it's a necessity that directly impacts your ability to provide compassionate, practical support to your loved ones or patients.

## The Impact of Self-Care on Caregiving Quality

The quality of care you provide is intrinsically linked to your well-being. When you prioritize self-care, you benefit yourself and enhance your capacity to care for others. Let's explore how self-care positively influences various aspects of caregiving:

1. **Enhanced Emotional Resilience**
    - Better equipped to handle stress and emotional challenges
    - Increased patience and empathy in difficult situations
    - Improved ability to maintain a calm demeanor

2. **Improved Physical Stamina**
    - Greater energy to perform caregiving tasks
    - Reduced risk of caregiver-related injuries
    - Increased overall health, leading to fewer sick days

3. **Sharpened Mental Acuity**
    - Better decision-making skills in critical situations
    - Improved memory and attention to detail
    - Enhanced problem-solving abilities

4. **Strengthened Relationships**
    - more positive interactions with the care recipient

- Healthier boundaries with family members and healthcare professionals
- Improved communication skills

5. **Increased Caregiving Longevity**
    - Reduced risk of burnout and compassion fatigue
    - Sustained ability to provide care over extended periods
    - Greater job satisfaction for professional caregivers

| Self-Care Practice | Benefits to Caregiver | Impact on Caregiving Quality |
|---|---|---|
| **Regular Exercise** | Improved physical health, stress relief | Increased energy, better mood during care |
| **Adequate Sleep** | Better cognitive function, emotional stability | Enhanced decision-making, patience in care |
| **Mindfulness/Meditation** | Reduced anxiety, improved focus | Increased presence and empathy in interactions |
| **Social Connections** | Emotional support, reduced isolation | Renewed energy and perspective in caregiving |

# Overcoming Guilt and Prioritizing Personal Needs

One of the most significant barriers to self-care for caregivers is the pervasive feeling of guilt. It's common to feel that taking time for yourself is selfish or detracts from the care you should provide. However, overcoming this guilt is essential for sustainable caregiving. Here's how to reframe your thinking and prioritize your needs:

**Understanding Guilt in Caregiving:**

- Recognize that guilt is a common and normal emotion for caregivers
- Acknowledge that guilt often stems from unrealistic expectations of yourself
- Realize that neglecting your needs can lead to resentment and diminished care quality

**Strategies for Overcoming Caregiver Guilt:**

1. **Reframe Your Perspective**
   - View self-care as a necessary part of providing good care
   - Understand that taking care of yourself allows you to be more present and effective
   - Recognize that you're modeling healthy behavior for others

2. **Set Realistic Expectations**
   - Accept that you can't do everything perfectly
   - Understand that it's okay to have limits and boundaries
   - Recognize that asking for help is a sign of strength, not weakness

3. **Practice Self-Compassion**
   - Treat yourself with the same kindness you show to others
   - Acknowledge your efforts and successes, no matter how small
   - Use positive self-talk to counter guilty thoughts

4. **Educate Yourself and Others**
    - Learn about the importance of self-care in caregiving literature
    - Share information with family members to gain their support
    - Discuss the benefits of caregiver well-being with healthcare professionals

5. **Start Small and Build**
    - Begin with short periods of self-care to ease into the practice
    - Gradually increase the time and frequency of self-care activities
    - Celebrate each step you take towards prioritizing your needs

**Practical Steps to Prioritize Personal Needs:**

- **Schedule Self-Care**: Block out time in your calendar for activities that rejuvenate you
- **Create a Self-Care Plan**: Develop a written plan outlining your self-care goals and strategies
- **Communicate Your Needs**: Clearly express your needs to family members and support networks
- **Use Respite Care**: Take advantage of respite services to get regular breaks
- **Join Support Groups**: Connect with other caregivers who understand your challenges
- **Seek Professional Help**: Consider therapy or counseling to work through feelings of guilt

| Common Guilt-Inducing Thoughts | Reframed Perspective |
|---|---|
| "I should be doing more." | "I'm doing my best, and that's enough." |
| "Taking a break is selfish." | "Taking care of myself helps me provide better care." |
| "Nobody else can care for them like I can." | "Accepting help allows for fresh energy in caregiving." |
| "I don't deserve to enjoy myself." | "My well-being is important and valid." |

Remember, prioritizing your needs isn't selfish—it's essential. You can continue providing the high-quality, compassionate care that your loved ones or patients deserve by taking care of yourself. Self-care is integral to the caregiving journey, benefiting you and those you care for. Embrace it without guilt, knowing that you're making a wise investment in your ability to care for others.

# Physical Self-Care Strategies

Your physical health is the foundation of your ability to provide care as a caregiver. While putting your needs last is easy, maintaining your physical well-being is crucial for you and your loved one. Let's explore practical strategies to keep your body healthy and energized.

## Maintaining a Healthy Diet

A nutritious diet is essential for sustaining your energy levels and overall health. Here are some strategies to ensure you're fueling your body properly:

1. **Plan and Prepare Meals in Advance**
    - Use weekends or less busy times to batch-cook meals
    - Freeze portions for easy reheating during hectic days
    - Prepare healthy snacks to avoid reaching for processed foods

2. **Focus on Nutrient-Dense Foods**

- o Incorporate a variety of colorful fruits and vegetables
- o Choose whole grains over refined carbohydrates
- o Include lean proteins like fish, poultry, beans, and nuts
- o Don't forget healthy fats from sources like avocados and olive oil

3. **Stay Hydrated**
   - o Keep a water bottle with you throughout the day
   - o Set reminders to drink water regularly
   - o Include hydrating foods like cucumbers and watermelon in your diet

4. **Mindful Eating**
   - o Take time to sit down and enjoy your meals
   - o Avoid eating while multitasking or when stressed
   - o Listen to your body's hunger and fullness cues

5. **Seek Support**
   - o Ask family members or friends to help with meal preparation
   - o Consider meal delivery services for fresh, healthy options
   - o Consult a nutritionist for personalized dietary advice if needed

| Meal Type | Quick and Healthy Options |
|---|---|
| Breakfast | Greek yogurt with berries and nuts, overnight oats, whole grain toast with avocado. |
| Lunch | Mixed green salad with grilled chicken, whole grain wrap with hummus and vegetables. |
| Dinner | Baked salmon with roasted vegetables, vegetarian chili, stir-fry with tofu and mixed veggies. |
| Snacks | Apple slices with almond butter, carrot sticks with hummus, and a handful of mixed nuts. |

## Incorporating Regular Exercise

Exercise is not just about physical fitness; it's a powerful stress reliever and mood booster. Here's how to make physical activity a regular part of your routine:

1. **Find Activities You Enjoy**
    - Experiment with different types of exercise to find what you like
    - Consider activities that can involve your loved one, like gentle walks
    - Try yoga or tai chi for both physical and mental benefits

2. **Set Realistic Goals**
    - Start small. Even 10 minutes a day can make a difference
    - Gradually increase duration and intensity as you build stamina
    - Celebrate your progress, no matter how small

3. **Make It Convenient**
    - Keep exercise equipment at home for quick workouts
    - Use online fitness videos for guided sessions
    - Take advantage of small pockets of time throughout the day

4. **Incorporate Movement into Daily Tasks**
    - Do calf raises while washing dishes
    - Perform stretches during TV commercials
    - Take the stairs instead of the elevator when possible

5. **Seek Support and Accountability**
    - Join a caregiver fitness group or online community
    - Use fitness apps to track your progress
    - Ask a friend or family member to be your exercise buddy

| Exercise Type | Benefits | Caregiver-Friendly Examples |
| --- | --- | --- |
| Cardiovascular | Improves heart health, boosts energy | Brisk walking, dancing, stationary cycling |
| Strength Training | Builds muscle, supports bone health | Bodyweight exercises, resistance bands, light dumbbells |
| Flexibility | Reduces muscle tension, improves mobility | Gentle stretching, yoga, tai chi |
| Balance | Prevents falls, improves stability | Single-leg stands, heel-to-toe walk, balance board |

# Ensuring Adequate Sleep and Rest

Quality sleep is crucial for your physical and mental well-being. Here are strategies to improve your sleep habits:

1. **Establish a Consistent Sleep Schedule**
    - Try to go to bed and wake up at the same time each day
    - Create a relaxing bedtime routine to signal your body it's time to sleep
    - Avoid screens for at least an hour before bedtime

2. **Optimize Your Sleep Environment**
    - Keep your bedroom cool, dark, and quiet
    - Invest in a comfortable mattress and pillows
    - Use white noise or earplugs if needed to block out disturbances

3. **Manage Nighttime Caregiving**
    - Use night lights to avoid fully waking up for nighttime checks
    - Consider assistive devices like bed alarms to alert you when needed
    - Take turns with other family members for nighttime care if possible

4. **Practice Relaxation Techniques**
    - Try deep breathing exercises before bed
    - Use guided imagery or meditation to calm your mind
    - Practice progressive muscle relaxation to release physical tension

5. **Be Mindful of Diet and Exercise**
    - Avoid caffeine and heavy meals close to bedtime
    - Exercise regularly, but not too close to bedtime
    - Limit alcohol, as it can disrupt sleep patterns
6. **Prioritize Rest During the Day**
    - Take short power naps (15-20 minutes) when possible
    - Use respite care to get a whole night's sleep occasionally
    - Practice mindfulness or meditation for mental rest during the day

| Sleep Challenge | Potential Solution |
| --- | --- |
| **Difficulty falling asleep** | Practice a calming bedtime routine, and try relaxation techniques. |
| **Waking up during the night** | Keep a notepad by your bed to jot down thoughts, and use white noise. |
| **Early morning wakings** | Ensure your room is dark, and consider adjusting your sleep schedule. |
| **Feeling unrested after sleep** | Evaluate your sleep environment and consult a doctor about sleep quality. |

Remember, taking care of your physical health is not selfish—it's a necessary part of being an effective caregiver. By prioritizing your diet, exercise, and sleep, you're ensuring you have the strength and energy to provide the best care possible for your loved one. Start with small, manageable changes, and be patient with yourself as you develop these healthy habits. Your body—and your loved one—will thank you for it.

# Emotional and Mental Well-being

As a caregiver, tending to your emotional and mental health is just as crucial as maintaining your physical well-being. The demands of caring for a loved one can significantly toll your psychological state, making it essential to develop strategies that nurture your inner self. Let's explore some effective methods to support your emotional and mental well-being.

## Practicing Mindfulness and Meditation

Mindfulness and meditation are powerful tools for managing stress, improving focus, and cultivating inner peace. These practices can be particularly beneficial for caregivers, offering moments of calm in challenging situations.

**Benefits of Mindfulness and Meditation for Caregivers:**

- Reduced stress and anxiety
- Improved emotional regulation
- Enhanced ability to focus and concentrate
- Increased self-awareness and empathy
- Better sleep quality
- Boosted immune function

**How to Incorporate Mindfulness and Meditation into Your Daily Routine:**

1. **Start Small**
    - Begin with just 5 minutes a day
    - Gradually increase the duration as you become more comfortable

2. **Choose a Consistent Time and Place**
    - Set aside a specific time each day for your practice
    - Create a quiet, comfortable space for meditation

3. **Explore Different Techniques**
   - Try guided meditations using apps or online resources
   - Experiment with breathing exercises, body scans, or loving-kindness meditation
   - Practice mindful activities like walking or eating

4. **Be Patient and Non-Judgmental**
   - Remember that it's normal for your mind to wander
   - Gently bring your attention back to your focus point without self-criticism

5. **Integrate Mindfulness into Daily Activities**
   - Practice being fully present during routine tasks like washing dishes or folding laundry
   - Take mindful breaks throughout the day, even if just for a few deep breaths

| Mindfulness Technique | Description | When to Use |
| --- | --- | --- |
| **Breath Awareness** | Focus on the sensation of breathing, noticing each inhale and exhale | Any time, especially during stressful moments |
| **Body Scan** | Systematically relax each part of your body from head to toe | Before bed or during breaks |
| **Loving-Kindness Meditation** | Direct positive thoughts and wishes towards yourself and others | When feeling overwhelmed or frustrated |
| **Mindful Walking** | Pay attention to each step and your surroundings while walking | During outdoor breaks or while moving between tasks |

# Journaling and Emotional Expression

Journaling is a powerful tool for processing emotions, gaining clarity, and fostering self-reflection. For caregivers, it can serve as a private outlet for expressing the complex feelings often accompanying caregiving.

**Benefits of Journaling for Caregivers:**

- Emotional release and stress reduction
- Increased self-awareness and problem-solving
- Documentation of caregiving journey and memories
- Opportunity for a gratitude practice
- Improved communication skills

**Tips for Effective Journaling:**

1. **Choose Your Medium**
    - Traditional pen and paper
    - Digital journaling apps or word processors
    - Audio recordings or voice memos

2. **Set Aside Regular Time**
    - Aim for consistency, even if it's just a few minutes daily
    - Choose a time when you're least likely to be interrupted

3. **Write Freely Without Judgment**
    - Don't worry about grammar, spelling, or structure
    - Let your thoughts flow without censoring yourself

4. **Use Prompts When Needed**
    - "Today, I felt..."
    - "I'm grateful for..."
    - "A challenge I faced today was..."
    - "Something I learned about myself is..."
5. **Reflect on Your Entries**
    - Periodically review your journal to observe patterns and growth
    - Use insights gained to inform your self-care and caregiving strategies
6. **Explore Different Journaling Techniques**
    - Gratitude journaling
    - Stream of consciousness writing
    - Dialogue journaling (writing conversations with yourself or others)
    - Art journaling (combining writing with visual elements)

| Journaling Method | Description | Benefit for Caregivers |
| --- | --- | --- |
| Gratitude Journal | Daily list of things you're thankful for | Shifts focus to positive aspects of caregiving |
| Emotional Release Writing | Unfiltered expression of feelings and thoughts | Helps process difficult emotions and experiences |
| Problem-Solving Journal | Writing out challenges and brainstorming solutions | Enhances coping skills and decision-making |
| Reflection Journal | Regular entries about personal growth and insights | Promotes self-awareness and resilience |

# Seeking Professional Mental Health Support

While self-care practices are essential, there may be times when professional support is necessary. Seeking help from a mental health professional is a sign of strength and can provide valuable tools for managing the emotional challenges of caregiving.

**Signs You May Benefit from Professional Support:**

- Persistent feelings of sadness, anxiety, or hopelessness
- Difficulty managing anger or frustration
- Feeling overwhelmed or unable to cope
- Changes in sleep patterns or appetite
- Loss of interest in activities you once enjoyed
- Thoughts of self-harm or suicide

**Types of Professional Mental Health Support:**

1. **Individual Therapy**
    - One-on-one sessions with a licensed therapist or counselor.
    - Can focus on specific caregiving challenges or broader emotional issues.

2. **Support Groups**
    - Facilitated groups for caregivers to share experiences and coping strategies.
    - It can be in-person or online.

3. **Cognitive Behavioral Therapy (CBT)**
    - It helps identify and change negative thought patterns and behaviors.
    - It is particularly effective for managing anxiety and depression.

4. **Mindfulness-Based Stress Reduction (MBSR)**
    - Combines mindfulness meditation and yoga to reduce stress.
    - Often offered in 8-week programs.

5. **Telehealth Options**
    - Virtual therapy sessions via video call or phone.
    - Convenient for caregivers with limited time or transportation.

**Steps to Access Mental Health Support:**

1. **Consult Your Primary Care Physician**
    - Discuss your concerns and get referrals to mental health professionals.

2. **Check with Your Insurance Provider**
    - Understand your coverage for mental health services.
    - Get a list of in-network providers.

3. **Research Local Resources**
    - Contact local hospitals or community centers for caregiver support programs.
    - Look into non-profit organizations specializing in your loved one's condition.

4. **Consider Online Platforms**
    - Explore reputable online therapy services.
    - Look for platforms that offer specific support for caregivers.

5. **Don't Hesitate to Try Different Options**
    - Switching therapists is okay if you don't feel a good connection.
    - Explore different types of therapy to find what works best for you.

| Type of Support | Best For | Potential Drawbacks |
|---|---|---|
| Individual Therapy | Personalized attention, deep exploration of issues | It can be costly, time-consuming |
| Support Groups | Shared experiences, practical advice from peers | Less individual focus and may not address specific needs |
| Online Therapy | Convenience, flexibility in scheduling | Potential technology issues, less personal connection |
| Crisis Hotlines | Immediate support during acute stress or emergencies | Not suitable for ongoing, in-depth support |

Remember, taking care of your emotional and mental well-being is not a luxury—it's a necessity. By practicing mindfulness, journaling, and seeking professional support when needed, you're investing in your ability to provide compassionate care. Be patient with yourself as you explore these strategies, and remember that it's okay to prioritize your mental health. A mentally healthy caregiver is better equipped to face the challenges of caregiving with resilience and grace.

## Building a Support Network

As a caregiver, it's crucial to remember that you don't have to face this journey alone. Building a solid support network can provide emotional support, practical assistance, and valuable resources. Let's explore how you can create and nurture a network that will sustain you through the challenges of caregiving.

# Joining Caregiver Support Groups

Caregiver support groups offer a unique opportunity to connect with others who truly understand your experiences. These groups can be invaluable sources of emotional support, practical advice, and camaraderie.

**Benefits of Joining Caregiver Support Groups:**

- Emotional validation and understanding
- Sharing of practical tips and resources
- Reduced feelings of isolation and loneliness
- Opportunity to help others and feel empowered
- Access to educational resources and expert speakers

**Types of Caregiver Support Groups:**

1. **In-Person Groups**
    - Often held at community centers, hospitals, or religious organizations
    - Provide face-to-face interaction and immediate support

2. **Online Forums and Groups**
    - Accessible from anywhere, at any time
    - Offer anonymity and convenience

3. **Condition-Specific Groups**
    - Focus on caregivers dealing with particular illnesses or conditions
    - Provide specialized information and understanding

4. **Demographic-Specific Groups**
    - Cater to specific caregiver demographics (e.g., spouses, adult children, young caregivers)
    - Address unique challenges faced by different caregiver populations

**How to Find and Join a Support Group:**

1. Research local options through hospitals, community centers, or disease-specific organizations
2. Explore online platforms like Facebook groups or caregiver-specific websites
3. Ask your healthcare provider for recommendations
4. Consider starting your group if you can't find one that meets your needs

| Type of Group | Pros | Cons |
| --- | --- | --- |
| **In-Person** | Personal connection, immediate support | Time commitment, transportation needed |
| **Online** | Convenient, accessible 24/7 | Lack of face-to-face interaction |
| **Condition-Specific** | Targeted advice, shared experiences | It may be limited in availability |
| **General Caregiver** | Broader perspective, diverse experiences | May lack specificity for your situation |

## Involving Family and Friends

Your existing network of family and friends can be a powerful source of support. However, many caregivers struggle with asking for help or feel guilty about burdening others. Remember, most people want to help but may not know how.

**Strategies for Involving Family and Friends:**

1. **Be Specific About Your Needs**
    - Create a list of tasks that others can help with
    - Be clear about what kind of support you're looking for (practical, emotional, etc.)

2. **Use Technology to Coordinate**
    - Utilize care coordination apps or shared calendars
    - Set up a group chat or email thread for updates and requests

3. **Educate Them About Your Caregiving Situation**
    - Share information about your loved one's condition
    - Help them understand the challenges you face

4. **Foster Ongoing Connections**
    - Schedule regular check-ins or social gatherings
    - Encourage friends and family to maintain a relationship with your care recipient

5. **Express Gratitude**
    - Thank helpers for their support, no matter how small
    - Let them know the positive impact of their assistance

**Overcoming Barriers to Asking for Help:**

- Recognize that accepting help benefits both you and your care recipient
- Start small if you're uncomfortable asking for big favors
- Remember that people often want to help but don't know how

| Practice asking for help to become more comfortable with it Type of Support | Examples | How to Ask |
|---|---|---|
| Practical Assistance | Meal preparation, house cleaning, errands | "Could you pick up groceries for us this week?" |
| Respite Care | Sitting with the care recipient, overnight care | "Can you stay with Mom for a few hours on Saturday?" |
| Emotional Support | Listening, checking in, offering encouragement | "I'm having a tough week. Could we chat over coffee?" |
| Financial Help | Assistance with bills, fundraising | "We're struggling with medical expenses. Can you help us set up a fundraiser?" |

# Utilizing Community Resources and Respite Care

Community resources and respite care services can provide crucial support, allowing you to take breaks and access specialized assistance. These resources can help prevent burnout and ensure better care for you and your loved one.

**Types of Community Resources:**

1. **Area Agencies on Aging (AAA)**
    - Provide information, referrals, and sometimes direct services
    - Often offer caregiver support programs and resources

2. **Local Senior Centers**
   - May offer adult daycare programs
   - Provide social activities and meals for seniors

3. **Faith-Based Organizations**
   - Often have volunteer programs to assist caregivers
   - May offer support groups or counseling services

4. **Non-Profit Organizations**
   - Condition-specific organizations often have local chapters with resources
   - May offer educational workshops, support groups, or financial assistance

**Respite Care Options:**

1. **In-Home Respite**
   - Professional caregivers come to your home
   - Can range from a few hours to overnight care

2. **Adult Day Centers**
   - Provide care and activities during daytime hours
   - Often include meals and social interaction for care recipients

3. **Residential Respite**
   - Short-term stays at assisted living facilities or nursing homes
   - Allows for extended breaks or travel

4. **Volunteer Respite Programs**
   - Often run by community organizations or faith groups
   - May offer limited hours of free care

**Steps to Access Community Resources and Respite Care:**

1. Contact your local AAA for a comprehensive list of resources
2. Speak with your loved one's healthcare provider for recommendations
3. Research condition-specific organizations for specialized support
4. Explore online directories of senior services and respite care options
5. Consult with a social worker or case manager for personalized guidance

| Resource Type | Services Offered | How to Access |
| --- | --- | --- |
| Area Agency on Aging | Information, referrals, caregiver support programs | Call the local office or visit the website |
| Adult Day Centers | Daytime care, activities, meals | Contact the center directly for a tour and assessment |
| Home Health Agencies | In-home care, nursing services, respite | Get a referral from a doctor or contact an agency |
| Volunteer Programs | Companionship, errands, light housekeeping | Contact local senior centers or faith organizations |

Remember, building a strong support network is an ongoing process. Finding the right combination of support groups, family involvement, and community resources that work for you may take time. Be patient with yourself and persistent in seeking out the help you need. By creating a robust support system, you're taking care of yourself and ensuring you can provide the best possible care for your loved one.

Don't hesitate to reach out and accept help when it's offered. Your role as a caregiver is invaluable, and by taking care of yourself through building a strong support network, you're ensuring that you can continue to provide compassionate care for the long term.

## Time Management and Organization

As a caregiver, you often juggle multiple responsibilities, making time management and organization crucial skills. Effective planning can help reduce stress, increase efficiency, and ensure you and your loved one receive the care and attention needed. Let's explore strategies to help you manage your time and effectively organize your caregiving duties.

## Creating a Caregiving Schedule

A well-structured caregiving schedule can provide a sense of routine and predictability, which benefits both you and your care recipient. Here's how to create an effective caregiving schedule:

1. **Assess Care Needs**
   - List all daily, weekly, and monthly tasks required for your loved one's care.
   - Include medical appointments, medication times, and personal care routines.

2. **Prioritize Tasks**
   - Identify critical tasks that must be done at specific times.
   - Determine which tasks are flexible and can be rescheduled if needed.

3. **Create a Template**
   - Use a digital calendar or a large paper calendar.
   - Color-code different types of activities for easy visualization.

4. **Include Self-Care**
   - Schedule time for your appointments, breaks, and activities.
   - Block out time for sleep and regular meals.

5. **Be Realistic**
    - Allow extra time for tasks, as caregiving often takes longer than expected.
    - Build buffer time for unexpected events or emergencies.
6. **Review and Adjust Regularly**
    - Reassess the schedule weekly or monthly.
    - Make changes as care needs evolve or your situation changes.

| Time | Task | Responsible Person |
|---|---|---|
| 7:00 AM | Morning medications and breakfast | Primary Caregiver |
| 9:00 AM | Personal care and dressing | Home Health Aide |
| 11:00 AM | Physical therapy exercises | Primary Caregiver |
| 1:00 PM | Lunch and afternoon medications | Family Member |
| 3:00 PM | Social activity or rest | Volunteer Companion |
| 6:00 PM | Dinner and evening medications | Primary Caregiver |
| 8:00 PM | Bedtime routine | Primary Caregiver |

# Delegating Tasks and Accepting Help

Delegating tasks and accepting help are essential for maintaining your well-being and ensuring comprehensive care for your loved one. Here's how to approach delegation effectively:

1. **Identify Delegable Tasks**
    - Make a list of tasks that don't require your specific expertise.
    - Consider which tasks others might enjoy or be well-suited to perform.

2. **Match Tasks to Helpers**
   - Consider the skills, availability, and preferences of potential helpers.
   - Assign tasks that align with each person's strengths and schedules.

3. **Communicate Clearly**
   - Provide detailed instructions for each task.
   - Set clear expectations for how and when tasks should be completed.

4. **Express Appreciation**
   - Thank helpers for their contributions, no matter how small.
   - Acknowledge the positive impact of their assistance.

5. **Be Open to Different Methods**
   - Recognize that others may complete tasks differently than you would.
   - Focus on results rather than specific methods when possible.

6. **Overcome Reluctance to Delegate**
   - Remind yourself that accepting help benefits both you and your loved one.
   - Start small if you're uncomfortable with extensive delegation.

**Strategies for Effective Delegation:**
- Use a shared task list or care coordination app.
- Rotate responsibilities among family members.
- Consider hiring professional help for specialized tasks.
- Utilize volunteer services for non-medical assistance.

| Task Category | Examples | Potential Delegates |
|---|---|---|
| Household Chores | Cleaning, laundry, yard work | Family members, hired help, volunteers |
| Errands | Grocery shopping, pharmacy runs | Friends, neighbors, delivery services |
| Personal Care | Bathing, dressing, grooming | Home health aides, trained family members |
| Social Support | Companionship, activities | Friends, volunteers, adult day programs |
| Medical Management | Medication reminders, doctor appointments | Nursing services, tech solutions, family members |

# Using Technology to Streamline Caregiving Duties

Technology can be a powerful ally in managing caregiving responsibilities. Various tools can help simplify your caregiving journey, from organizing tasks to monitoring health. Here's how to leverage technology effectively:

1. **Care Coordination Apps**

    o Use apps designed for caregivers to manage schedules, tasks, and communication.

    o Examples: Caring Village, Lotsa Helping Hands, and CaringBridge.

2. **Medication Management Tools**

    o Utilize apps or smart pill dispensers to track and remind about medications.

    o Consider: Medisafe, PillPack, and Hero.

3. **Health Monitoring Devices**
    - Implement wearable devices or smart home sensors for health tracking.
    - Options: Fall detection devices, blood pressure monitors, GPS trackers.

4. **Communication Tools**
    - Use video calling apps to connect with your loved one and other caregivers.
    - Try: Skype, FaceTime, or Zoom.

5. **Online Support and Education**
    - Access online forums, webinars, and caregiver support and education courses.
    - Explore: Family Caregiver Alliance, AARP Caregiver Resource Center.

6. **Smart Home Devices**
    - Implement voice-activated assistants and smart home technology for added convenience and safety.
    - Consider: Amazon Alexa, Google Home, smart thermostats, and automated lighting.

**Tips for Implementing Caregiving Technology:**

- Start with one or two tools and gradually add more as needed.
- Ensure all caregivers are trained on how to use the technology.
- Regularly review and update your tech tools as care needs change.
- Consider the comfort level of your care recipient with technology.

| Technology Type | Benefits | Considerations |
| --- | --- | --- |
| Care Coordination Apps | Improved communication, task management | Requires all caregivers to adopt and use consistently |
| Health Monitoring Devices | Early detection of health issues, increased independence | It may require professional setup, ongoing costs |
| Medication Management Tools | Reduced medication errors, improved adherence | Need for regular updates, potential tech glitches |
| Smart Home Devices | Enhanced safety, convenience for daily tasks | Initial setup cost, learning curve for usage |

Remember, effective time management and organization are ongoing processes. Be patient with yourself as you implement these strategies, and don't hesitate to adjust your approach as needed. You can create a more manageable and sustainable caregiving routine by creating a structured schedule, delegating tasks, and leveraging technology.

These tools and strategies are meant to support you, not add stress. Please choose the best methods for your unique situation and gradually incorporate them into your caregiving routine. With time and practice, you'll likely find that improved organization leads to more quality time with your loved one and better self-care for you as a caregiver.

## Maintaining Personal Identity and Interests

As a caregiver, it's easy to become so immersed in your responsibilities that you lose sight of your identity and interests. However, maintaining a sense of self is crucial for your well-being and can make you a more effective caregiver. Let's explore ways to nurture your identity and interests while balancing your caregiving duties.

## Pursuing Hobbies and Passions

Engaging in activities you enjoy is not a luxury—it's necessary to maintain your mental and emotional health. Here's how to keep your hobbies and passions alive:

1. **Identify Time Pockets**
    - Look for small windows of time in your schedule
    - Consider early mornings, during care recipient's naps, or after bedtime

2. **Adapt Your Hobbies**
    - Find ways to engage in your interests in shorter time frames
    - Look for portable versions of your hobbies

3. **Involve Your Care Recipient**
    - When possible, find ways to include your loved one in your activities
    - This can provide stimulation for them and enjoyment for you both

4. **Use Technology**
    - Explore online classes or virtual communities related to your interests
    - Use apps or online resources to engage in hobbies remotely

5. **Schedule Regular "Me Time"**
    - Block out time in your calendar for your interests
    - Treat this time as crucial as any other appointment

**Ideas for Maintaining Hobbies:**

- Reading: Join an online book club or use audiobooks during commutes
- Art: Keep a sketchbook for quick drawing sessions
- Music: Create playlists to enjoy while performing caregiving tasks
- Gardening: Start a small indoor herb garden or tend to potted plants
- Exercise: Try short workout videos or practice yoga during breaks

| Hobby Type | Adaptation for Caregivers | Benefits |
|---|---|---|
| Reading | E-books, audiobooks, short stories | Mental stimulation, stress relief |
| Crafting | Portable projects (knitting, sketching) | Creativity outlet, sense of accomplishment |
| Fitness | Short home workouts, walking | Physical health, energy boost |
| Cooking | Quick recipes, meal prep | Nutrition, enjoyment, potential involvement of care recipient |

## Staying Connected with Friends

Maintaining social connections is vital for your emotional well-being and provides a support system outside your caregiving role. Here are strategies to stay connected:

1. **Leverage Technology**
   - Use video calls, social media, or messaging apps to stay in touch
   - Join online groups or forums related to your interests

2. **Schedule Regular Check-ins**
   - Set up recurring phone calls or virtual coffee dates with friends
   - Use calendar reminders to prompt you to reach out
3. **Be Honest About Your Situation**
   - Share your caregiving challenges with trusted friends
   - Let them know how they can support you
4. **Plan for Social Activities**
   - Arrange respite care to allow for occasional outings
   - Invite friends for short visits at home when possible
5. **Involve Friends in Caregiving**
   - Ask friends to visit or spend time with your care recipient
   - This can provide you with a break while maintaining connections

**Tips for Maintaining Friendships:**

- Quality over quantity: Focus on nurturing a few close relationships
- Be present: When you do have time with friends, try to be fully engaged
- Share your caregiving journey: Allow friends to understand your life
- Accept help: Let friends support you in practical ways if they offer

| Connection Type | Ideas for Caregivers | Potential Challenges |
| --- | --- | --- |
| Virtual Meetups | Video chat coffee dates, online game nights | Technology issues, scheduling conflicts |
| In-Person Visits | Short home visits, park meetups | Limited time, need for care coverage |
| Group Activities | Book clubs, virtual workout groups | Finding common interests, time commitment |
| Caregiving Involvement | Friend visits with care recipient, help with tasks | Friends' comfort level with caregiving situation |

## Setting Personal Goals Outside of Caregiving

Setting and working towards personal goals can provide a sense of purpose and achievement beyond your caregiving role. Here's how to approach goal-setting:

1. **Reflect on Your Aspirations**
    - Think about what you want to achieve for yourself
    - Consider short-term and long-term goals
2. **Start Small**
    - Set realistic, achievable goals given your current situation
    - Break larger goals into smaller, manageable steps
3. **Make Goals SMART**
    - Specific, Measurable, Achievable, Relevant, Time-bound
    - This framework helps create clear, actionable goals

4. **Write Down Your Goals**
    - Use a journal or goal-tracking app to document your objectives
    - Regularly review and update your goals

5. **Seek Support**
    - Share your goals with friends or family who can encourage you
    - Consider finding an accountability partner

6. **Celebrate Progress**
    - Acknowledge and celebrate each step towards your goals
    - Use achievements as motivation to continue pursuing your aspirations

**Examples of Personal Goals for Caregivers:**

- Learning: Take an online course or learn a new language
- Health: Establish a regular exercise routine or improve eating habits
- Career: Maintain professional skills or explore part-time work options
- Creative: Start a blog, write a book, or create art
- Personal Growth: Practice mindfulness or develop a new skill

| Goal Category | Example Goal | Potential Steps |
|---|---|---|
| Education | Complete an online certificate program | Research programs, allocate study time, set completion date |
| Health and Wellness | Establish a regular meditation practice. | Download the app, start with 5 minutes daily, and gradually increase the time. |
| Personal Development | Improve time management skills. | Read productivity books, try a time-blocking technique, and use organization apps. |
| Creative Expression | Write and publish a short story | Set writing schedule, join writing group, research publishing options |

Remember, maintaining your identity and interests is not selfish—it's essential for your well-being and can make you a more effective and compassionate caregiver. By pursuing your hobbies, staying connected with friends, and setting personal goals, you're taking care of yourself and bringing fresh energy and perspective to your caregiving role.

Feeling guilty about taking time for yourself is normal, but remember that self-care is crucial to sustainable caregiving—your loved one benefits when you're refreshed, fulfilled, and connected to your identity. Be patient with yourself as you navigate this balance, and don't hesitate to adjust your approach as your caregiving situation evolves. Your growth and well-being are important to you and those you care for.

# Coping with Grief and Loss

As a caregiver, you may find yourself navigating complex emotions, including grief and loss, long before your loved one's passing. Understanding and addressing these feelings is crucial for your emotional well-being and ability to provide compassionate care. Let's explore how to cope with these challenging aspects of the caregiving journey.

# Acknowledging Anticipatory Grief

Anticipatory grief is the grief experienced before an impending loss. For caregivers, this can begin when a loved one is diagnosed with a progressive illness or when you start to notice significant declines. Recognizing and addressing this grief is an integral part of your emotional health.

**Signs of Anticipatory Grief:**

- Sadness or tearfulness
- Anxiety about the future
- Loneliness or isolation
- Anger or irritability
- Guilt or regret
- Physical symptoms like fatigue or changes in appetite

**Strategies for Coping with Anticipatory Grief:**

1. **Acknowledge Your Feelings**
    - Recognize that your grief is valid and normal
    - Allow yourself to experience and express your emotions

2. **Seek Support**
    - Join a caregiver support group
    - Consider talking to a therapist or counselor
    - Confide in trusted friends or family members

3. **Practice Self-Care**
    - Engage in activities that bring you comfort
    - Maintain your physical health through diet and exercise
    - Set aside time for relaxation and stress relief

4. **Create Meaningful Moments**
    - Make new memories with your loved one
    - Document your journey through journaling or photography
    - Engage in life review conversations with your loved one

5. **Educate Yourself**
    - Learn about your loved one's condition and what to expect
    - Understand the grief process and its various manifestations

| Emotion | Coping Strategy | Self-Care Action |
|---------|-----------------|------------------|
| **Sadness** | Allow yourself to cry; express emotions through art or writing | Practice gratitude journaling; spend time in nature |
| **Anxiety** | Use relaxation techniques; focus on the present moment | Try meditation or deep breathing exercises |
| **Guilt** | Challenge negative thoughts; practice self-compassion | Engage in positive self-talk; seek validation from support group |
| **Anger** | Find healthy outlets like exercise; communicate feelings assertively | Practice stress-relief techniques; consider counseling |

# Finding Meaning in the Caregiving Journey

While caregiving can be challenging, many find it offers opportunities for personal growth, deepened relationships, and a sense of purpose. Finding meaning in your caregiving role can help you cope with the difficulties and find moments of joy and fulfillment.

**Ways to Find Meaning in Caregiving:**

1. **Reflect on Your Values**
    - Consider how caregiving aligns with your values
    - Recognize the positive impact you're making in your loved one's life

2. **Practice Mindfulness**
    - Stay present in the moment, appreciating small joys
    - Use mindfulness techniques to manage stress and find peace

3. **Cultivate Gratitude**
    - Keep a gratitude journal, noting the positive aspects of each day
    - Share moments of appreciation with your loved one

4. **Learn and Grow**
    - View challenges as opportunities for personal development
    - Acquire new skills and knowledge through your caregiving role

5. **Connect with Others**
    - Share your experiences with other caregivers
    - Offer support and mentorship to those new to caregiving

6. **Create a Legacy Project**
    - Work with your loved one to create something meaningful (e.g., a memory book, video, or family history project)

| Aspect of Caregiving | Potential for Meaning | Action to Cultivate Meaning |
|---|---|---|
| Find ways to honor your loved one's life and values | | |
| Daily Care Tasks | Expressing love through service | Practice mindfulness during care routines |
| Emotional Support | Deepening relationship bonds | Engage in life review conversations |
| Learning New Skills | Personal growth and empowerment | Recognize and celebrate your growing expertise |
| Advocating for Loved One | Standing up for what's right | Reflect on how advocacy aligns with your values |

# Self-Advocacy and Setting Boundaries

As a caregiver for someone with dementia, you're often so focused on your loved one's needs that you might forget to advocate for yourself. Remember, your well-being is just as important. Let's explore how you can effectively communicate your needs, set boundaries, and maintain a healthy balance in your life.

## Communicating needs effectively

Effective communication is critical to meeting your needs while caring for someone with dementia. Here are some strategies to help you communicate more effectively:

1. Be clear and specific about your needs
2. Use "I" statements to express your feelings
3. Choose the right time and place for meaningful conversations
4. Practice active listening when others are speaking
5. Be open to compromise and negotiation

| Communication Do's | Communication Don'ts |
| --- | --- |
| **Express yourself calmly and respectfully.** | Use accusatory language or blame others. |
| **Be specific about what you need.** | Assume others know what you're thinking. |
| **Listen to others' perspectives.** | Interrupt or dismiss others' opinions. |
| **Take time to collect your thoughts.** | React impulsively when emotions are high. |

## Learning to say 'no' when necessary

As a caregiver, you may feel obligated to say 'yes' to every request or task related to your loved one's care. However, learning to say 'no' when necessary is crucial for your well-being and the quality of care you provide. Here's how you can start setting limits:

- Recognize your limits: Be honest about what you can realistically handle.
- Prioritize tasks: Focus on the most essential and remove less critical responsibilities.
- Practice saying 'no': Start small and work up to more significant boundaries.
- Offer alternatives: Suggest other solutions or resources if you can't do something.
- Don't feel guilty: Remember that setting boundaries is healthy and necessary.

## Balancing caregiving with other responsibilities

Striking a balance between caregiving and other aspects of your life can be challenging, but it's essential for your overall well-being. Here are some strategies to help you maintain equilibrium:

1. Create a schedule: Allocate time for caregiving, work, family, and personal activities.

2. Delegate tasks: Involve other family members or hire help for specific responsibilities.

3. Use respite care: Take advantage of short-term care options to give yourself a break.

4. Maintain your health: Prioritize your physical and mental well-being through regular check-ups and self-care.

5. Stay connected: Nurture relationships outside of your caregiving role.

| Area of Life | Strategies for Balance |
| --- | --- |
| Work | Discuss flexible options with your employer, and consider part-time work if possible. |
| Family | Schedule regular family time and involve children in age-appropriate caregiving tasks. |
| Personal Time | Set aside time each day for activities you enjoy, even if it's just for 15 minutes. |
| Social Life | Join a support group and plan regular outings with friends. |

Remember, caring for yourself isn't selfish—it's necessary. By advocating for your needs, setting boundaries, and maintaining balance in your life, you'll be better equipped to provide quality care for your loved one with dementia. Don't hesitate to seek support when you need it, whether from family, friends, or professional resources. You're doing important and challenging work and deserve care and support.

# Continuing Education and Skills Development

As a caregiver for someone with dementia, your journey is one of continuous learning and growth. Staying informed about the latest care techniques and developing your skills can significantly improve your loved one's quality of life and your caregiving experience. Let's explore how you can enhance your knowledge and abilities in this challenging but rewarding role.

## Staying informed about dementia care techniques

Dementia care is an evolving field, with new research and techniques emerging regularly. Keeping up-to-date with these developments can help you provide the best possible care for your loved one. Here are some ways to stay informed:

1. Subscribe to reputable dementia care newsletters
2. Follow leading dementia organizations on social media
3. Join online forums or support groups for caregivers
4. Read books and articles by dementia care experts
5. Consult regularly with healthcare professionals involved in your loved one's care

| Resource Type | Examples | Benefits |
| --- | --- | --- |
| **Newsletters** | Alzheimer's Association, Dementia Society of America | Regular updates on research and care techniques |
| **Online Forums** | Alzheimer's Association ALZConnected, Dementia Talking Point | Peer support and shared experiences |
| **Books** | "The 36-Hour Day" by Nancy L. Mace and Peter V. Rabins | In-depth knowledge and practical advice |

## Attending workshops and seminars

Workshops and seminars offer valuable opportunities to learn from experts, connect with other caregivers, and gain hands-on experience with new care techniques. Consider the following when seeking out educational opportunities:

- Look for local events hosted by hospitals, community centers, or dementia care organizations
- Explore online webinars and virtual conferences for convenient learning options

- Attend caregiver support group meetings that often feature educational components
- Investigate training programs offered by local hospice or home health agencies
- Consider certification programs in dementia care if you're looking for more comprehensive education

Remember, investing time in these educational opportunities benefits your loved one and is an act of self-care that can boost your confidence and reduce stress in your caregiving role.

## Developing patience and communication skills

Caring for someone with dementia requires extraordinary patience and effective communication skills. These abilities don't always come naturally but can be developed and improved over time. Here are some strategies to enhance these crucial skills:

1. Practice mindfulness and deep breathing to stay calm in challenging situations
2. Learn about the stages of dementia to better understand and anticipate your loved one's needs
3. Use non-verbal communication techniques, such as maintaining eye contact and using a gentle touch
4. Speak clearly and slowly, using simple language and short sentences
5. Develop strategies for redirecting and de-escalating challenging behaviors

| Skill | Importance | Development Strategies |
|---|---|---|
| **Patience** | Reduces stress and improves quality of care | Practice mindfulness, take regular breaks, seek support when needed |
| **Communication** | It enhances understanding and reduces frustration | Learn about non-verbal cues, practice active listening, and adjust your speaking style |
| **Empathy** | Builds trust and strengthens your relationship | Try to see situations from your loved one's perspective, and join a support group to share experiences. |

Developing these skills takes time and practice. Be patient with yourself as you learn and grow in your caregiving role. Remember that every caregiver faces challenges, and it's okay to make mistakes. What's important is your commitment to learning and improving.

By staying informed about dementia care techniques, attending educational events, and continually developing your patience and communication skills, you can improve your care and take important steps to prevent burnout and maintain your well-being.

Your dedication to learning and growing as a caregiver is admirable. It reflects the depth of your commitment to your loved one and personal growth. As you continue on this journey, remember that every new skill you acquire and every bit of knowledge you gain is a valuable tool in your caregiving toolkit, helping you navigate the challenges of dementia care with greater confidence and compassion.

# Planning: Legal and Financial Considerations

**Taking care of a loved one with dementia is a journey that requires both compassion and preparation.** As you embark on this path, addressing legal and financial matters early on is not just important; it's a responsibility. This proactive approach can save you from stress and complications, allowing you to focus on what truly matters - providing love and care for your loved one with dementia.

## Understanding the Importance of Early Planning

**Early planning is not just a precaution; it's a necessity.** When your loved one is in the early stages of dementia, they may still have the mental capacity to make crucial decisions and express their wishes. By addressing legal and financial matters early, you:

- Ensure your loved one's voice is heard in future care decisions
- Protect their assets and finances
- Reduce potential family conflicts
- Gain peace of mind for both you and your loved one

Remember, dementia is progressive. There may come a time when your family member can no longer make sound decisions or sign legal documents. **Acting early puts you in the best position to honor their wishes and manage their care effectively.**

# Financial and Legal Considerations

Navigating caregiving's financial and legal aspects can be overwhelming for a caregiver. However, understanding these elements is crucial for ensuring the best care for your loved one and protecting your financial well-being. Let's explore the key areas you need to consider.

## Planning for Long-Term Care Expenses

Long-term care can be costly, and planning to manage these expenses effectively is essential. Here are some steps to help you prepare:

1. **Assess Current and Future Needs**
   - Evaluate your loved one's current health status and potential future needs
   - Consider the possibility of in-home care, assisted living, or nursing home care

2. **Estimate Costs**
   - Research the costs of different care options in your area
   - Factor in potential increases in healthcare costs over time

3. **Review Available Resources**
   - Assess your loved one's savings, assets, and income sources
   - Consider potential family contributions

4. **Explore Insurance Options**
   - Look into long-term care insurance policies
   - Understand what Medicare and Medicaid may cover

5. **Consult Financial Professionals**
   - Speak with a financial advisor experienced in elder care planning
   - Consider meeting with an elder law attorney

**Long-Term Care Funding Options:**

- Personal savings and assets
- Long-term care insurance
- Life insurance policies with long-term care riders
- Reverse mortgages (for homeowners)

- Veterans benefits (for eligible veterans and their spouses)
- Medicaid (for those who qualify based on financial need)

| Care Type | Average Monthly Cost (2024) | Potential Funding Sources |
|---|---|---|
| In-Home Care (44 hours/week) | $4,000 - $8,000 | Personal funds, LTC insurance, Medicaid waivers |
| Assisted Living Facility | $4,500 - $7,000 | Personal funds, LTC insurance, some Medicaid programs |
| Nursing Home (Semi-Private Room) | $7,000 - $14,000 | Medicare (short-term), Medicaid, personal funds, LTC insurance |
| Nursing Home (Private Room) | $8,000 - $15,000 | Medicare (short-term), Medicaid, personal funds, LTC insurance |
| Adult Day Health Care | $1,800 - $2,600 | Medicaid waivers, personal funds, some LTC insurance policies |

# Understanding Legal Rights and Options

Navigating the legal aspects of caregiving is crucial for protecting your loved one's interests and ensuring their wishes are respected. Here are critical legal considerations:

1. **Advance Directives**
    - Encourage your loved one to create or update their advance directives
    - Ensure you have copies of living wills and healthcare power of attorney documents

2. **Power of Attorney**
    - Understand the difference between medical and financial power of attorney
    - Consider setting up a durable power of attorney for finances and healthcare

3. **Guardianship/Conservatorship**
    - Know when these might be necessary and how to pursue them if needed
    - Understand the responsibilities and limitations of these roles

4. **Estate Planning**
    - Encourage your loved one to create or update their will
    - Discuss options like trusts for managing assets

5. **HIPAA Authorization**
    - Ensure you have the necessary authorization to access your loved one's medical information

**Essential Legal Documents for Caregivers:**

- Durable Power of Attorney for Healthcare
- Durable Power of Attorney for Finances
- Living Will
- HIPAA Authorization Form
- Will and Trust Documents
- Do Not Resuscitate (DNR) Order (if applicable)

| Legal Document | Purpose | When to Obtain |
|---|---|---|
| Healthcare Power of Attorney | Designates someone to make medical decisions if the person is incapacitated | As early as possible while the person can make sound decisions |
| Financial Power of Attorney | Allows the designated person to manage finances | Before the cognitive decline, update as needed |
| Living Will | Specifies end-of-life care preferences | When creating advance directives, review them periodically |
| HIPAA Authorization | Allows access to medical information | When beginning the caregiving role, update annually |

# Medical Power of Attorney: What It Is and Why It Matters

A Medical Power of Attorney (MPOA) is a legal document that allows your loved one to appoint someone they trust to make healthcare decisions on their behalf if they cannot do so themselves. This person is often called a healthcare proxy or agent.

**Why is an MPOA crucial?**

1. It ensures medical decisions align with your loved one's wishes
2. It prevents potential disagreements among family members about care
3. It allows for quick decision-making in emergencies
4. It gives healthcare providers a clear point of contact for meaningful discussions

To set up an MPOA:

1. Discuss the role with your loved one and decide who should be the healthcare proxy
2. Consult with an elder law attorney to draft the document
3. Ensure the document is properly signed and witnessed
4. Provide copies to healthcare providers and family members

# Financial Power of Attorney: Protecting Assets and Finances

A Financial Power of Attorney (FPOA) is similar to an MPOA but focuses on financial matters. This document allows your loved one to designate someone to manage their finances if they cannot do so themselves.

**Critical aspects of an FPOA:**

- It can be immediate or "springing" (only taking effect under specific circumstances)
- It can be broad or limited in scope
- It ends upon the death of your loved one

**Benefits of having an FPOA:**

- Ensures bills are paid, and finances are managed properly
- Protects against financial exploitation
- Allows for long-term financial planning
- Provides a clear authority for financial institutions to work with

# Living Wills and Advance Directives

A living will, often part of an advance directive, is a document that outlines your loved one's wishes for end-of-life care. It typically covers preferences for:

- Use of life-sustaining treatments
- Pain management and comfort care
- Organ donation

**Why are these documents important?**

- They provide clear guidance in difficult situations
- They reduce the emotional burden on family members making tough decisions
- They ensure your loved one's wishes are respected, even if they can't communicate

# When and How to Have These Conversations

**Timing is crucial when discussing these sensitive topics.** Here are some tips:

1. Start early, ideally when your loved one is first diagnosed
2. Choose a calm, private setting
3. Include other family members if appropriate
4. Be patient and prepared for multiple conversations

**Conversation starters:**

- "I know this is hard to discuss, but I want to ensure we honor your wishes."
- "Have you thought about what kind of medical care you'd want if you couldn't make decisions?"
- "I've been reading about the importance of having certain legal documents. Can we talk about that?"

# Finding Legal Assistance for Document Preparation

While finding templates for these documents online is possible, **working with an elder law attorney is highly recommended.** They can:

- Ensure documents are correctly prepared and legally binding
- Provide advice on complex family or financial situations
- Help navigate state-specific laws and requirements

To find a qualified attorney:

- Ask for recommendations from your local Alzheimer's Association chapter
- Contact your state or local bar association
- Look for attorneys certified in elder law by the National Elder Law Foundation

**Proper legal preparation can save significant future stress, time, and money.**

| Document | Purpose | Key Points |
|---|---|---|
| Medical Power of Attorney | Designates someone to make healthcare decisions | • Choose a trusted individual<br>• Discuss preferences in advance<br>• Provide copies to healthcare providers |
| Financial Power of Attorney | Allows someone to manage finances | • Can be immediate or "springing"<br>• Protects against financial exploitation<br>• Ends upon death |
| Living Will/Advance Directive | Outlines end-of-life care preferences | • Covers life-sustaining treatments<br>• Addresses pain management<br>• Includes organ donation wishes |

By addressing these legal and financial considerations early, you're taking a crucial step in ensuring the best possible care for your loved one with dementia. Remember, you're not alone in this journey. Seek support from professionals, support groups, and your community as you navigate this challenging but essential process.

# Exploring Financial Assistance Programs

Various programs and resources are available to help ease the financial burden of caregiving. Here's an overview of potential assistance options:

1. **Government Programs**
    - Medicare: Understand coverage for hospital stays, doctor visits, and some home healthcare
    - Medicaid: Explore eligibility for long-term care coverage
    - Social Security Disability Insurance (SSDI): For those under 65 with qualifying disabilities
    - Supplemental Security Income (SSI): For low-income individuals with disabilities

2. **Veterans Benefits**
    - Aid and Attendance benefits for veterans and surviving spouses
    - Veteran-Directed Care Program
    - VA Caregiver Support Program

3. **State and Local Programs**
    - Area Agencies on Aging: Local resources and support programs
    - State-specific caregiver support programs
    - Respite care grants or vouchers

4. **Non-Profit Organizations**
    - Disease-specific organizations offering financial assistance
    - Local charities and community organizations

5. **Employer Benefits**
    - Check if your employer offers caregiver support or flexible work arrangements
    - Employee Assistance Programs (EAPs) may provide counseling or referrals

6. **Tax Deductions and Credits**
    - Explore potential tax benefits for caregivers
    - Consult a tax professional to understand your eligibility

**Steps to Access Financial Assistance:**

1. Research programs you might be eligible for
2. Gather necessary documentation (medical records, financial information)
3. Contact program administrators or local offices for application procedures
4. Consider seeking help from a social worker or case manager to navigate options
5. Be persistent and don't hesitate to appeal if initially denied

| Assistance Type | Potential Programs | Eligibility Factors |
| --- | --- | --- |
| Government Assistance | Medicare, Medicaid, SSDI, SSI | Age, disability status, income, assets |
| Veterans Benefits | Aid and Attendance, VA Caregiver Support | Military service, disability rating, income |
| State Programs | Caregiver support, respite care grants | Varies by state, often based on need |
| Non-Profit Assistance | Disease-specific org grants, local charities | Diagnosis, financial need, location |

Remember, navigating caregiving's financial and legal aspects can be complex, but you don't have to do it alone. Don't hesitate to seek professional advice from financial advisors, elder law attorneys, or social workers specializing in senior care. Many communities offer free or low-cost legal clinics and financial counseling services for caregivers.

Addressing these matters early and revisiting them regularly as circumstances change is essential. By understanding and planning for caregiving's financial and legal aspects, you can ensure better care for your loved one and protect your financial well-being.

Understanding and managing these considerations can provide peace of mind, allowing you to focus more energy on the day-to-day aspects of caregiving and your relationship with your loved one. Remember, being proactive in these areas is an integral part of your role as a caregiver and a vital aspect of self-care.

# Validation Therapy

## Naomi Feil's Validation Therapy

Validation Therapy is a compassionate approach developed by Naomi Feil to help people with dementia feel understood and valued. It involves acknowledging and validating their feelings and experiences rather than trying to correct or dismiss them.

### History and Development

Naomi Feil, a social worker, developed validation therapy between 1963 and 1980. She grew up in a family home for seniors and noticed that traditional therapies often upset or isolated elderly patients with dementia. She sought a better way to communicate with them, leading to the creation of Validation Therapy.

**Key milestones:**

- **1963-1980:** Development of Validation Therapy by Naomi Feil
- **1982:** Publication of Feil's first book on Validation Therapy
- **1980s:** Gained attention in the U.S. through presentations and research

### Core Principles

Validation Therapy is based on several core principles guiding caregivers' interactions with dementia patients.

**Core principles include:**

1. **Acceptance:** Accept the person where they are and where they are not.
2. **Empathy:** Step into their world and feel what they feel.
3. **Respect:** Validate their emotions and experiences without judgment.
4. **Communication:** Use verbal and non-verbal techniques to connect.

| Principle | Description |
| --- | --- |
| Acceptance | Accept the person as they are |
| Empathy | Feel what they feel. |
| Respect | Validate emotions and experiences. |
| Communication | Use verbal and non-verbal techniques. |

## Benefits for Dementia Patients

Validation Therapy offers numerous benefits for dementia patients, helping them feel more connected and less isolated.

**Benefits include:**

- **Restoration of self-worth:** Patients feel valued and understood.
- **Reduced withdrawal:** Encourages interaction with others.
- **Decreased stress and anxiety:** Provides emotional comfort.
- **Improved communication:** Enhances the ability to express feelings.
- **Stimulation of potential:** Helps patients engage in meaningful activities.

| Benefit | Description |
| --- | --- |
| Restoration of self-worth | Patients feel valued and understood. |
| Reduced withdrawal | Encourages interaction with others |
| Decreased stress and anxiety | Provides emotional comfort |
| Improved communication | Enhances ability to express feelings |
| Stimulation of potential | Helps patients engage in meaningful activities |

# Techniques and Examples

Validation Therapy uses specific techniques to connect with dementia patients and validate their feelings.

**Techniques include:**

- **Mirroring:** Reflecting the patient's body language and emotions.
- **Rephrasing:** Restating what the patient says to show understanding.
- **Reminiscence:** Encouraging patients to talk about past experiences.
- **Touch:** Using gentle touch to convey empathy and support.
- **Eye contact:** Maintaining eye contact to build trust.

**Examples of techniques:**

1. **Mirroring:**
    - If a patient is wringing their hands, the caregiver might gently mimic this action to show empathy.

2. **Rephrasing:**
    - Patient: "I need to find my mother."
    - Caregiver: "You miss your mother and want to see her."

3. **Reminiscence:**
    - Asking the patient about their favorite childhood memory.

4. **Touch:**
    - Holding the patient's hand during a conversation.

5. **Eye contact:**
    - Looking into the patient's eyes while speaking to them.

| Technique | Example |
| --- | --- |
| **Mirroring** | Mimicking hand-wringing to show empathy |
| **Rephrasing** | "You miss your mother and want to see her." |
| **Reminiscence** | Asking about favorite childhood memory |
| **Touch** | Holding the patient's hand |
| **Eye contact** | Maintaining eye contact during conversation |

Using these techniques, caregivers can create a supportive and understanding environment for dementia patients, helping them feel more secure and less anxious. Validation Therapy is a powerful tool that respects the dignity and emotions of those with dementia, fostering meaningful connections and improving their overall well-being.

# Other Validation Techniques

In addition to Naomi Feil's Validation Therapy, several other nonpharmacological methods can be effective in managing dementia symptoms. These methods focus on empathetic communication and creating a supportive environment for dementia patients.

## Empathetic Listening

Empathetic listening involves genuinely hearing and understanding what the person with dementia is saying verbally and non-verbally.

**Steps for empathetic listening:**

1. **Be present:** Give your full attention to the person.

2. **Acknowledge feelings:** Reflect on what you hear to show understanding.

3. **Avoid judgment:** Accept their feelings without trying to correct them.

4. **Use non-verbal cues:** Nod, maintain eye contact, and use appropriate facial expressions.

**Example:**

- Patient: "I feel so lost."

- Caregiver: "It sounds like you're feeling confused and scared. I'm here with you."

# Reassurance and Comfort

Providing reassurance and comfort can help alleviate fear and anxiety in dementia patients.

**Ways to provide reassurance:**

- **Verbal reassurance:** Use calming and soothing words.
- **Physical comfort:** Offer a gentle touch or a hug.
- **Familiar objects:** Provide comfort items, like a favorite blanket or photo.

**Example:**

- Patient: "I can't find my way home."
- Caregiver: "You're safe here with me. Let's sit together and talk."

# Reminiscence Therapy

Reminiscence therapy involves encouraging dementia patients to talk about their past experiences. This can help them feel more connected and valued.

**Benefits of reminiscence therapy:**

- **Improves mood:** Talking about happy memories can boost spirits.
- **Enhances communication:** Encourages verbal expression.
- **Strengthens identity:** Helps patients remember who they are.

**Techniques for reminiscence therapy:**

- **Use photos:** Show old family photos and ask about the people and events in them.
- **Music:** Play songs from their youth and discuss memories associated with the music.
- **Objects:** Use familiar objects to trigger memories and conversations.

**Example:**

- Caregiver: "Do you remember this photo from your wedding day? Tell me about that day."

## Reality Orientation

Reality orientation involves gently reminding dementia patients of the current time, place, and situation to help reduce confusion.

**Techniques for reality orientation:**

- **Use calendars and clocks:** Place them in visible locations.
- **Daily routines:** Maintain consistent daily schedules.
- **Verbal reminders:** Gently remind them of the date, time, and location.

**Example:**

- Caregiver: "Good morning, it's Tuesday, June 22nd. We're at home, and it's time for breakfast."

## Distraction and Redirection

Distraction and redirection involve shifting the patient's focus from distressing thoughts or behaviors to something more positive.

**Techniques for distraction and redirection:**

- **Engage in activities:** Suggest a favorite hobby or task.
- **Change the environment:** Move to a different room or walk.
- **Use humor:** Light-hearted jokes or funny stories can help.

**Example:**

- Patient: "I need to go to work."
- Caregiver: "Let's take a walk in the garden first. Look at these beautiful flowers!"

## Cognitive Stimulation Therapy

Cognitive Stimulation Therapy (CST) involves engaging dementia patients in activities that stimulate thinking and memory.

**Benefits of CST:**

- **Improves cognitive function:** Helps maintain mental abilities.
- **Enhances social interaction:** Encourages group activities and communication.
- **Boosts mood:** Engaging in activities can reduce depression and anxiety.

**Examples of CST activities:**

- **Puzzles and games:** Crosswords, Sudoku, and memory games.
- **Arts and crafts:** Painting, drawing, and crafting.
- **Group discussions:** Talking about current events or shared interests.

**Example:**

- Caregiver: "Let's work on this puzzle together. Can you find the corner pieces?"

# Environmental Modifications

Modifying the environment can help reduce confusion and agitation in dementia patients.

**Tips for environmental modifications:**

- **Simplify the space:** Remove clutter and unnecessary items.
- **Use clear signage:** Label rooms and essential items.
- **Ensure safety:** Install grab bars, remove tripping hazards, and use nightlights.

**Example:**

- Caregiver: "I've labeled the bathroom door and put a nightlight in the hallway to help you find your way at night."

| Technique | Description | Example |
|---|---|---|
| Empathetic Listening | Genuinely hearing and understanding the patient | "It sounds like you're feeling confused and scared. I'm here with you." |
| Reassurance and Comfort | Providing verbal and physical comfort | "You're safe here with me. Let's sit together and talk." |
| Reminiscence Therapy | Encouraging talk about past experiences | "Do you remember this photo from your wedding day? Tell me about that day." |
| Reality Orientation | Gently reminding of the current time, place, and situation | "Good morning, it's Tuesday, June 22nd. We're at home, and it's time for breakfast." |
| Distraction and Redirection | Shifting the focus to something positive | "Let's take a walk in the garden first. Look at these beautiful flowers!" |
| Cognitive Stimulation Therapy | Engaging in activities that stimulate thinking | "Let's work on this puzzle together. Can you find the corner pieces?" |
| Environmental Modifications | Modifying the environment to reduce confusion | "I've labeled the bathroom door and put a nightlight in the hallway to help you find your way at night." |

By using these nonpharmacological methods, caregivers can create a supportive and understanding environment for dementia patients, helping them feel more secure and less anxious. These techniques respect the dignity and emotions of those with dementia, fostering meaningful connections and improving their overall well-being.

# Practical Strategies for Caregivers

Caring for someone with dementia can be challenging, but with the right strategies, you can significantly improve their quality of life. Let's explore some practical approaches to help you provide the best care possible.

## Identifying and Addressing Unmet Needs

People with dementia may struggle to communicate their needs, leading to frustration and behavioral issues. You can often prevent or reduce challenging behaviors by identifying and addressing these unmet needs.

**Common unmet needs to look out for:**

- Physical discomfort (pain, hunger, thirst)
- Emotional distress (loneliness, boredom, anxiety)
- Environmental factors (too hot, too cold, too noisy)
- Need for routine or structure

**Steps to identify and address unmet needs:**

1. **Observe closely:** Watch for changes in behavior or mood.
2. **Keep a log:** Note patterns in behavior and potential triggers.
3. **Check for physical discomfort:** Ensure basic needs (food, water, toileting) are met.
4. **Offer comfort:** Provide reassurance and emotional support.
5. **Adjust the environment:** Make changes to reduce stress or discomfort.

| Need | Possible Signs | Potential Solutions |
|---|---|---|
| Hunger/Thirst | Agitation, wandering | Offer snacks or drinks regularly |
| Pain | Grimacing, guarding a body part | Consult with a doctor for pain management |
| Boredom | Restlessness, repetitive behaviors | Engage in meaningful activities |
| Overstimulation | Agitation, trying to leave | Create a calm, quiet space |

# Creating a Safe and Stable Environment

A safe and stable environment can significantly reduce anxiety and confusion for someone with dementia.

**Tips for creating a safe environment:**

- **Remove hazards:** Clear clutter, secure loose rugs, and remove dangerous items.
- **Enhance visibility:** Use contrasting colors for essential objects and improve lighting.

- **Simplify the space:** Reduce unnecessary furniture and decorations.

- **Use labels:** Clearly label essential rooms and items.

- **Maintain consistency:** Keep furniture arrangements stable and routines predictable.

**Creating a dementia-friendly home:**

1. **Kitchen:** Lock up hazardous items and use appliances with automatic shut-off features.

2. **Bathroom:** Install grab bars, use non-slip mats, and consider a raised toilet seat.

3. **Bedroom:** Ensure a clear path to the bathroom, and use nightlights.

4. **Living areas:** Remove or secure items that could cause trips or falls.

# Communication Tips for De-escalating Fear

Effective communication is critical to managing fear and anxiety in someone with dementia.

**General communication tips:**

- Speak clearly and slowly
- Use simple language and short sentences
- Maintain eye contact and a calm demeanor
- Use a gentle touch when appropriate

**Strategies for de-escalating fear:**

1. **Validate feelings:** Acknowledge their emotions without judgment.
    - Example: "I can see you're feeling scared. It's okay, I'm here with you."
2. **Use distraction:** Redirect attention to a pleasant topic or activity.
    - Example: "Let's look at your family photo album together."
3. **Provide reassurance:** Offer comfort and support.
    - Example: "You're safe here. I'll stay with you until you feel better."
4. **Create a calm environment:** Reduce noise and distractions.
    - Example: Turn off the TV, close curtains, or move to a quieter room.
5. **Use visual cues:** Show, don't just tell.
    - Example: If it's time for a meal, show them the table set with food.

**De-escalation techniques:**

| Technique | Description | Example |
| --- | --- | --- |
| Validation | Acknowledge feelings | "I understand you're feeling upset." |
| Distraction | Redirect attention | "Would you like to help me fold these towels?" |
| Reassurance | Provide comfort | "You're safe here with me." |
| Environment | Create calm | Reduce noise, adjust lighting |
| Visual cues | Show, don't tell | Point to or show objects instead of just describing them |

Remember, every person with dementia is unique, and what works for one may not work for another. Be patient, flexible, and willing to try different approaches. Your compassion and understanding can make a world of difference in the life of someone with dementia.

# Case Studies and Real-Life Examples

Understanding how different approaches work in real-life situations can be incredibly helpful for caregivers. Here, we will explore success stories with Validation Therapy and how combining pharmacological and nonpharmacological approaches can be effective.

**Success Stories with Validation Therapy**

Validation Therapy has been used successfully in many cases to improve the quality of life for dementia patients. Here are a few examples:

**Case Study 1: Mrs. Johnson**

**Background:**

- Mrs. Johnson, an 85-year-old woman with Alzheimer's disease, frequently called out for her deceased mother, causing distress to herself and her caregivers.

**Approach:**

- Caregivers used Validation Therapy by acknowledging her feelings and gently engaging her in conversations about her mother.

**Outcome:**

- Mrs. Johnson became calmer and more content. She started sharing happy memories about her mother, which reduced her anxiety and agitation.

**Case Study 2: Mr. Smith**

**Background:**

- Mr. Smith, a 78-year-old man with Lewy body dementia, often saw imaginary animals in his room, leading to fear and confusion.

**Approach:**

- Caregivers used Validation Therapy by acknowledging his fear and gently redirecting his attention to a favorite activity, like listening to music.

**Outcome:**

- Mr. Smith's episodes of fear decreased, and he became more engaged in activities he enjoyed, improving his overall mood.

| Case Study | Background | Approach | Outcome |
| --- | --- | --- | --- |
| Mrs. Johnson | Called out for deceased mother | Acknowledged feelings, engaged in conversations about mother | Reduced anxiety and agitation |
| Mr. Smith | Saw imaginary animals | Acknowledged fear, redirected to a favorite activity | Decreased fear, improved mood |

By using these nonpharmacological methods, caregivers can create a supportive and understanding environment for dementia patients, helping them feel more secure and less anxious. These techniques respect the dignity and emotions of those with dementia, fostering meaningful connections and improving their overall well-being.

# Navigating Placement
## Recognizing When More Care Is Needed

Caring for a loved one with dementia is an evolving journey. As the condition progresses, you may notice changes that signal a need for additional support. It's important to recognize these signs early to ensure the best care for your loved one and to protect your well-being.

### Signs That Home Care May No Longer Be Sufficient

**It's natural to want to keep your loved one at home for as long as possible, but there may come a time when home care is no longer enough.** Here are some signs to watch for:

- Increasing safety concerns (frequent falls, wandering, leaving appliances on)
- Difficulty managing daily tasks (bathing, dressing, eating)
- Incontinence issues that are hard to manage at home
- Aggressive or unpredictable behavior
- Sundowning syndrome (increased confusion and agitation in the evening)
- Caregiver exhaustion or inability to meet care needs

If you notice several of these signs, it may be time to consider additional care options.

### Assessing Safety Risks in the Home

**A safe home environment is crucial for someone with dementia.** As the condition progresses, what was once a safe space may become hazardous. Here's a checklist to help you assess potential risks:

- ☐ Remove or secure trip hazards like loose rugs or clutter
- ☐ Install handrails in bathrooms and on stairs
- ☐ Ensure good lighting throughout the house

- ☐ Lock away potentially dangerous items (medications, cleaning supplies, sharp objects)
- ☐ Consider safety devices like bed alarms or door sensors
- ☐ Remove or disable potentially dangerous appliances
- ☐ Adjust water heater temperature to prevent scalding

Remember, what seems obvious to you may not be clear to someone with dementia. Regular safety checks are essential.

## Caregiver Stress and Burnout: Recognizing Your Limits

**Caregiver burnout is a real and serious condition.** It's crucial to recognize the signs early to protect both your health and your ability to provide care. Watch for these symptoms:

- Feeling overwhelmed or constantly worried
- Feeling tired often
- Getting too much sleep or not enough sleep
- Gaining or losing weight
- Becoming easily irritated or angry
- Losing interest in activities you used to enjoy
- Feeling sad
- Having frequent headaches, bodily pain, or other physical problems
- Abusing alcohol or drugs, including prescription medications

If you're experiencing several of these symptoms, it's time to seek help. Remember, caring for yourself is not selfish—providing the best care for your loved one is necessary.

## The Importance of Regular Medical Evaluations

**Regular medical check-ups are vital for the person with dementia and the caregiver.** These evaluations can:

1. Monitor the progression of dementia

2. Identify and address new health issues early
3. Adjust medications as needed
4. Provide an opportunity to discuss care challenges
5. Offer recommendations for additional support or services

For the caregiver, regular health check-ups can:

1. Monitor stress levels and mental health
2. Address physical health concerns
3. Provide resources for caregiver support

**Don't hesitate to schedule appointments more frequently if you notice changes or have concerns.**

| Aspect of Care | Warning Signs | Possible Solutions |
| --- | --- | --- |
| Safety | Frequent falls, wandering, unsafe use of appliances | Home modifications, safety devices, increased supervision |
| Personal Care | Difficulty with bathing, dressing, eating | In-home care assistance, adaptive equipment |
| Behavior | Aggression, severe mood swings, sundowning | Medication review, behavior management strategies, professional care |
| Caregiver Health | Exhaustion, depression, neglecting own health | Respite care, support groups, considering facility care |

Remember, recognizing the need for more care doesn't mean you've failed. It means you're making a responsible decision to ensure the best possible quality of life for your loved one and yourself. Every situation is unique, and there's no one-size-fits-all solution. Trust your instincts, communicate with healthcare providers, and don't be afraid to ask for help when needed.

# Understanding Care Facility Options

When caring for a loved one with dementia becomes challenging at home, it's essential to understand the various care facility options available. Each type of facility offers different levels of care and services to meet the unique needs of individuals with dementia.

## Types of Care Facilities: An Overview

Three main types of care facilities cater to individuals with dementia:

1. Assisted Living Facilities
2. Memory Care Units
3. Skilled Nursing Facilities

Each of these options provides a different level of care and support. Let's explore them in more detail.

## Assisted Living Facilities: What They Offer

**Assisted Living Facilities (ALFs) bridge independent living and nursing home care.** They offer a combination of housing, personal care services, and health care designed to assist individuals with regular daily activities.

Services typically offered in ALFs include:

- Help with activities of daily living (bathing, dressing, eating)
- Medication management
- Housekeeping and laundry services
- Meals and dining support
- Social and recreational activities
- Transportation services

ALFs are an excellent option for individuals who:

- Need more personal care services than can be provided at home
- Are still relatively independent but require some assistance

- Don't need the intensive medical care provided in a nursing home

## Memory Care Units: Specialized Care for Dementia

**Memory Care Units are specifically designed to meet the needs of individuals with Alzheimer's disease and other forms of dementia.** These units are often part of an assisted living facility or nursing home, but some are stand-alone.

Key features of Memory Care Units include:

- Secure environments to prevent wandering
- Specially trained staff in dementia care
- Activities tailored to enhance cognitive function
- Structured routines to reduce confusion and anxiety
- Design elements to aid in navigation and reduce overstimulation

Memory Care Units are ideal for individuals who:

- Have mid to late-stage dementia
- require a higher level of care and supervision
- Need a secure environment due to wandering behaviors
- Benefit from specialized dementia care programming

## Skilled Nursing Facilities: When More Medical Care Is Needed

**Skilled Nursing Facilities (SNFs), or nursing homes, provide the highest level of care outside of a hospital.** They offer 24-hour supervised care, including medical care and support services.

Services provided in SNFs include:

- 24-hour nursing care
- Rehabilitation services (physical, occupational, and speech therapy)
- Assistance with all activities of daily living

- Medication management
- Nutritional support and meal services
- Social services and recreational activities

SNFs are appropriate for individuals who:

- Require round-the-clock medical supervision
- Have complex medical needs in addition to dementia
- Need extensive assistance with daily activities
- Require post-hospital or post-surgery care

## Comparing Costs and Services Across Facility Types

When considering care options, comparing the services and associated costs is essential. Here's a general comparison:

| Facility Type | Level of Care | Average Monthly Cost* | Typically Covered By |
|---|---|---|---|
| Assisted Living | Low to Moderate | $4,500 to $7,000 | Private pay, some long-term care insurance |
| Memory Care | Moderate to High | $6,000 to $9,000 | Private pay, some long-term care insurance |
| Skilled Nursing | High | $7,000 to $15,000 | Medicare (short-term), Medicaid, private pay |

*Costs are national averages and can vary significantly by location and specific facility.

**When comparing facilities, consider:**

- The specific needs of your loved one
- The quality of care provided
- The facility's staff-to-resident ratio*
- The environment and available amenities
- The location and accessibility for family visits
- The cost and payment options available

*It is common for facility administrators and marketing staff to include staff with titles who, in theory, can provide direct patient care but sit at a desk and do not participate in care. For example, a facility may have an intake position where the person holds a certified nursing assistant (CNA) certificate or a licensed practical nurse (LPN) where the person holds a nursing license and yet provides no actual direct care. A skilled nursing facility often has a medical records person with a registered nursing license (RN) who provides no direct care. By incorporating these additional persons into the staff ratios, they can appear to be better prepared to care for loved ones within the facility than their competition and make it look like they have appropriate staffing for the State Department of Health. When you ask about staff-to-resident ratios, be particular about the staff on the floor who do not have "desk jobs."

Remember, the best choice depends on your loved one's needs, your family's resources, and the options available in your area. It's often helpful to visit multiple facilities and speak with staff, current residents, or their families before deciding.

Choosing a care facility is a significant decision, and feeling overwhelmed is normal. Don't hesitate to seek guidance from healthcare providers, social workers, or elder care specialists who can provide personalized advice based on your situation.

# Financial Considerations for Long-Term Care

Planning for long-term care can feel overwhelming, especially concerning finances. Understanding your options and available resources is crucial to making informed decisions for your loved one's care.

# Estimating the Costs of Different Care Options

**Long-term care costs can vary widely depending on the type of care and your location.** Here's a general overview of average monthly costs in the United States:

| Type of Care | Average Monthly Cost |
| --- | --- |
| In-Home Care | $4,000 - $8,000 |
| Assisted Living | $4,500 - $7,000 |
| Memory Care | $6,000 - $9,000 |
| Nursing Home (Semi-Private Room) | $7,000 - $14,000 |
| Nursing Home (Private Room) | $8,000 - $15,000 |

Remember, these are national averages. Costs can be significantly higher or lower depending on your specific location and the level of care needed.

To estimate costs in your area:

1. Research local facilities and in-home care agencies
2. Request detailed pricing information
3. Consider additional costs like medications, personal items, and specialized care

# Understanding Long-Term Care Insurance

**Long-term care insurance can help cover care costs, but it's essential to understand how it works.**

Key points about long-term care insurance:

- It typically covers care not covered by health insurance, Medicare, or Medicaid
- Policies vary widely in what they cover and for how long
- The best time to purchase is when you're younger and healthier
- Premiums can be expensive and may increase over time

- There's usually a waiting period before benefits kick in

If you're considering long-term care insurance:

- Compare policies from multiple providers
- Understand precisely what is and isn't covered
- Consider your family health history and potential care needs
- Consult with a financial advisor to determine if it's right for you

## Veterans Benefits for Long-Term Care

**If your loved one is a veteran, they may be eligible for long-term care benefits through the Department of Veterans Affairs (VA).**

VA long-term care benefits may include:

- Nursing home care
- Residential settings providing personal care services
- Home health care
- Adult day health care
- Respite care

Eligibility depends on several factors:

1. Service-connected disability status
2. Income level
3. Ability to perform daily living activities
4. Available VA resources

To explore VA benefits:

1. Contact your local VA office
2. Speak with a VA benefits counselor
3. Visit the VA website for detailed information

# Introduction to Medicaid for Long-Term Care

**Medicaid is a joint federal and state program that can help cover long-term care costs for eligible individuals.**

*Medicaid Eligibility Criteria*

Medicaid eligibility is based on both financial and functional needs. While criteria can vary by state, general requirements include:

Financial Criteria:

- Limited income (typically up to 300% of the SSI federal benefit rate)
- Limited assets (often around $2,000 for an individual, excluding certain protected assets)

Functional Criteria:

- Need assistance with activities of daily living (bathing, dressing, eating, etc.)
- Require a nursing home level of care

*The Medicaid Application Process*

Applying for Medicaid can be complex. Here's a general overview of the process:

1. Gather necessary documentation (financial, medical, etc.)
2. Complete the Medicaid application form
3. Apply to your local Medicaid office
4. Undergo a functional assessment to determine the level of care needs
5. Await the decision (can take 45-90 days)
6. If approved, work with Medicaid to set up care

**Important:** Medicaid examines all financial transactions for a five-year "look-back" period. Improper transfers during this time can result in penalties.

*Where to Get Help with Medicaid Applications*

Navigating the Medicaid application process can be challenging. Consider seeking help from:

- Elder law attorneys specializing in Medicaid planning
- Geriatric care managers
- Local Area Agency on Aging offices
- Medicaid planning professionals
- Social workers at local hospitals or senior centers

**Remember:** Rules and processes can vary by state. Always consult with professionals familiar with your state's specific Medicaid program.

Planning for long-term care finances is a complex process, but you don't have to navigate it alone. Don't hesitate to seek professional advice to ensure you make the best decisions for your loved one's care and your family's financial well-being.

# Choosing the Right Facility

Selecting the proper care facility for your loved one is a significant decision that requires careful consideration. This process can feel overwhelming, but breaking it down into steps can make it more manageable. Let's explore how to approach this critical choice.

## Assessing Your Loved One's Specific Needs

**Before you start researching facilities, it's crucial to understand your loved one's needs.** This assessment will help narrow your options and ensure the chosen facility can provide appropriate care.

Consider the following aspects:

- Level of assistance needed with daily activities (bathing, dressing, eating)
- Medical needs (medication management, chronic condition care)
- Cognitive impairment level and related behaviors
- Mobility issues and fall risk

- Social and emotional needs
- Personal preferences and lifestyle

Create a list of these needs to refer to as you evaluate different facilities.

## Researching Facilities: What to Look For

Once you have a clear picture of your loved one's needs, start researching facilities in your area.

Key factors to consider include:

- Type of care provided (assisted living, memory care, skilled nursing)
- Facility size and layout
- Staff-to-resident ratio
- Specialized programs for dementia care
- Safety features and security measures
- Cleanliness and overall environment
- Reputation and ratings
- Cost and payment options

**Use online resources, ask for recommendations, and create a shortlist of facilities to visit in person.**

## Questions to Ask During Facility Tours

Visiting potential facilities is a crucial step in the decision-making process. Here's a list of essential questions to ask during your tours:

1. What types of care and services are provided?
2. How do you handle medical emergencies?
3. What is your staff turnover rate?
4. How do you manage challenging behaviors associated with dementia?
5. What is your policy on family involvement in care decisions?

6. Can residents bring personal belongings to make their space feel like home?
7. What activities and programs do you offer?
8. How do you ensure residents' safety and prevent wandering?
9. What is your medication management policy?
10. How do you communicate with families about their loved one's care?

## Understanding Staffing Ratios and Qualifications

**The quality of care your loved one receives is directly related to the staff providing that care.** Understanding staffing ratios and qualifications is crucial.

Key points to consider:

- Staff-to-resident ratio during day and night shifts
- Qualifications and training of staff members
- Presence of specialized memory care staff
- Availability of medical professionals (nurses, doctors)
- Staff turnover rate

A good facility should be transparent about their staffing information and willing to discuss it in detail.

## Evaluating Activities and Quality of Life Programs

**Engaging activities and programs are essential for maintaining the quality of life in a care facility.** Look for facilities that offer:

- Diverse daily activities tailored to residents' abilities and interests
- Programs that promote cognitive stimulation
- Physical exercise appropriate for residents' abilities
- Opportunities for social interaction
- Activities that involve music, art, or other creative pursuits

- Outdoor spaces and activities when possible

Ask for an activity calendar and observe residents participating in activities during your visit.

## Considering Location and Accessibility for Family Visits

The facility's location can significantly impact your ability to visit and stay involved in your loved one's care. Consider:

- Distance from your home or workplace
- Ease of transportation to the facility
- Parking availability
- Visiting hours and policies
- Options for private family gatherings within the facility

Remember, regular visits can significantly enhance your loved one's quality of life and allow you to monitor their care.

| Aspect to Consider | Questions to Ask |
|---|---|
| Care Needs | Can the facility meet all of my loved one's specific care needs? |
| Staff | What is the staff-to-resident ratio? What are staff qualifications? On any given day, how many resident care assistants or certified nursing assistants are providing care for how many residents? How many licensed personnel are on the floor at any one time providing direct care for how many residents? |
| Activities | What types of activities are offered? How often? |
| Safety | What safety measures are in place, especially for wandering? |
| Family Involvement | How can family members stay involved in care? |
| Cost | What is the total cost? What services are included? |

Choosing a care facility is a significant decision, and it's normal to feel mixed emotions during this process. Take your time, trust your instincts, and don't hesitate to ask for help or guidance. Remember, the goal is to find a place where your loved one will receive excellent care and maintain the best possible quality of life.

# Navigating Facility Admissions

Moving a loved one into a care facility can feel overwhelming. Understanding the steps involved and being prepared can help make this transition smoother for everyone involved.

## Understanding Admission Criteria

**Each facility has its own set of admission criteria.** These criteria help ensure that the facility can meet your loved one's needs and that they will be a good fit for the community. Common admission criteria include:

- Level of care needed
- Cognitive status
- Behavioral considerations
- Medical conditions and stability
- Ability to pay for care

During this process, it's essential to be honest about your loved one's needs and challenges. This will ensure they receive appropriate care and help avoid potential issues later.

## Required Documentation and Assessments

Facilities typically require a variety of documents and assessments before admission. While specifics may vary, you can generally expect to need:

Medical Documentation:

- Recent physical exam results
- List of current medications
- Immunization records

- Medical history and diagnoses

Legal Documentation:

- Power of attorney documents
- Advanced directives
- Medicare and Medicaid cards
- Social Security card

Financial Documentation:

- Proof of income
- Bank statements
- Insurance policies

Assessments:

- Cognitive assessment
- Functional assessment (ability to perform daily living activities)
- Behavioral assessment

**Having these documents organized in advance can significantly speed up the admission process.**

## Financial Considerations: Private Pay vs. Medicaid

Understanding payment options is crucial when navigating facility admissions.

Private Pay:

- Typically required for assisted living and many memory care units
- Allows for more choice in facilities
- Can be expensive long-term

Medicaid:

- Primarily covers nursing home care
- Has strict eligibility requirements based on income and assets

- May limit facility choices but can provide long-term financial support

Some facilities offer a "spend-down" option, where residents can transition to Medicaid once their private funds are depleted. **Be sure to discuss these options with the facility and understand their policies.**

| Payment Type | Pros | Cons |
| --- | --- | --- |
| **Private Pay** | More facility options, Often higher quality of care | It can be costly and may deplete savings quickly |
| **Medicaid** | Covers long-term care costs, No risk of running out of funds | Strict eligibility requirements, Limited facility choices |

## Negotiating Contracts and Understanding Fine Print

**Before signing any agreements, reviewing and understanding all contract terms is crucial.** Consider the following:

1. Review the contract carefully or have a lawyer review it
2. Understand all fees and what services they cover
3. Ask about potential rate increases and how they're determined
4. Clarify policies on room changes or level of care changes
5. Understand the conditions under which a resident might be asked to leave
6. Know the process for terminating the contract if needed

Don't hesitate to ask questions or request clarification on any points you don't understand. It's better to address these issues upfront than to face surprises later.

## Planning for the Move: A Checklist

Moving can be stressful, especially for someone with dementia. Here's a checklist to help make the transition smoother:

Before the Move:

- ☐ Sort through belongings, deciding what to bring
- ☐ Arrange for packing and moving assistance if needed
- ☐ Label all items being moved to the facility
- ☐ Inform family and friends of the upcoming move
- ☐ Cancel or redirect mail and services

Preparing the New Space:

- ☐ Visit the new room/apartment beforehand if possible
- ☐ Plan the layout of furniture and belongings
- ☐ Bring familiar items to create a sense of home
- ☐ Consider safety modifications if needed

Day of Move:

- ☐ Have all required documents ready
- ☐ Bring a supply of medications
- ☐ Pack a "first-night" bag with essentials
- ☐ Plan to stay with your loved one for a while to help them settle

After the Move:

- ☐ Help establish a routine
- ☐ Visit regularly, especially in the first few weeks
- ☐ Stay in communication with staff about how your loved one is adjusting
- ☐ Be patient – adjustment can take time

**Remember, feeling a range of emotions during this process is normal.** Give yourself and your loved one time to adjust. The goal is to ensure your family member receives the care they need in a safe and supportive environment.

# Enhancing Home Care When Facility Placement Isn't an Option

Caring for a loved one with dementia at home can be challenging, but with the right strategies and support, it's possible to provide excellent care while maintaining your well-being. Let's explore ways to enhance home care when facility placement isn't an option.

## Maximizing Safety in the Home Environment

**Creating a safe home environment is crucial for your loved one's well-being and peace of mind.** Consider these safety measures:

- Install handrails in bathrooms and on stairs
- Remove or secure tripping hazards like loose rugs
- Use locks on cabinets containing potentially dangerous items
- Install safety devices like stove shut-off systems
- Ensure good lighting throughout the house
- Consider a medical alert system

Regularly reassess the home environment as your loved one's needs change.

## Creating a Comprehensive Care Plan

A comprehensive care plan helps address your loved one's needs. Include:

1. Daily care routines (bathing, dressing, meals)
2. Medication management
3. Physical activity and exercise
4. Cognitive stimulation activities
5. Social engagement opportunities
6. Safety precautions
7. Emergency procedures

Review and update the care plan regularly with input from healthcare providers.

## Building a Support Network: Family, Friends, and Community Resources

**You don't have to do this alone.** Building a strong support network is essential for sustainable home care. Consider:

- Family members who can help with care or errands
- Friends who can provide companionship or respite
- Local support groups for caregivers
- Community services like Meals on Wheels
- Religious or spiritual communities
- Professional caregiving services for additional support

Remember, accepting help is a sign of strength, not weakness.

## Exploring Adult Day Care and Respite Services

Adult daycare and respite services can provide much-needed breaks for caregivers while ensuring your loved one is well-cared for. Benefits include:

- Social interaction with your loved one
- Structured activities and cognitive stimulation
- Time for caregivers to rest or attend to personal needs
- Opportunity to maintain employment while caregiving

Research local options and consider a trial period to see how your loved one responds.

## Utilizing Home Health and Hospice Services

Home health and hospice services can provide professional support in the home setting:

Home Health Services:

- Skilled nursing care

- Physical, occupational, or speech therapy
- Medical social services

Hospice Services:

- Pain and symptom management
- Emotional and spiritual support
- Respite care
- Bereavement support for families

**These services can be invaluable in managing complex care needs and enhancing quality of life.**

## Technology and Assistive Devices for Home Care

Technology can play a significant role in improving home care:

| Technology/Device | Purpose |
| --- | --- |
| Medication reminders | Ensure timely medication administration. |
| GPS trackers | Help locate a person who may wander. |
| Smart home devices | Control lighting, temperature, and security |
| Video monitoring | Allow remote check-ins |
| Fall detection systems | Alert caregivers to potential falls |

While technology can be helpful, it's important to balance its use with privacy considerations.

## Self-Care for Family Caregivers: Maintaining Your Well-being

**Taking care of yourself is not selfish – providing the best care for your loved one is necessary.** Prioritize self-care through:

1. Regular breaks and respite care
2. Maintaining your health appointments

3. Engaging in stress-reducing activities (exercise, meditation, hobbies)
4. Joining a support group or seeking counseling
5. Getting adequate sleep
6. Eating a healthy diet
7. Setting realistic expectations and boundaries

Remember the airplane oxygen mask analogy: You need to take care of yourself first to care for others effectively., but remember that.

Caring for a loved one with dementia at home is a journey that requires patience, flexibility, and support. Feeling overwhelmed is normal, but remember you're doing important and meaningful work. Don't hesitate to reach out for help when you need it, whether from family, friends, or professional services. Your well-being is just as important as your loved one's care.

# Making the Decision: Emotional and Practical Considerations

The decision to move a loved one with dementia into a care facility is often one of the most challenging choices a family can face. It's a process filled with complex emotions and practical considerations. Let's explore how to navigate this difficult journey.

## Dealing with Guilt and Mixed Emotions

**It's completely normal to experience a range of emotions when considering facility care for your loved one.** These may include:

- Guilt
- Relief
- Sadness
- Anxiety
- Grief

Remember, these feelings are a natural part of the process. Here are some strategies to cope:

1. Acknowledge your feelings without judgment
2. Remind yourself that seeking help is an act of love
3. Focus on the quality of care your loved one will receive
4. Share your feelings with trusted friends or a support group
5. Consider speaking with a therapist or counselor

**Remember, choosing facility care doesn't mean you've failed or that you love your family member any less.**

## Involving Your Loved One in the Decision-Making Process

It's essential to involve your loved one in decision-making when possible. This can help maintain their sense of autonomy and may ease the transition. Consider these approaches:

- Have open, honest conversations about care needs and options
- Visit potential facilities together if possible
- Ask for their input on what's important to them in a living environment
- Respect their preferences as much as possible within the constraints of their care needs
- If cognitive impairment is severe, focus on non-verbal cues and past expressed wishes

Remember, the goal is to honor your loved one's dignity while ensuring their safety and well-being.

## Family Dynamics: Navigating Disagreements About Care

Disagreements about care decisions are expected in families. Here are some strategies to navigate these challenges:

1. Schedule a family meeting to discuss care options

2. Encourage open, respectful communication
3. Focus on your loved one's needs rather than personal preferences
4. Consider involving a neutral third party, like a social worker or family therapist
5. Be willing to compromise and find creative solutions
6. Document decisions and plans to avoid future misunderstandings

**Remember, you're all on the same team, working towards the best care for your loved one.**

## Transitioning to New Roles: From Primary Caregiver to Advocate

Moving your loved one to a facility doesn't end your caregiving role—it transforms it. Your new role as an advocate is crucial. Here's how to transition effectively:

- Educate yourself about your loved one's rights in a care facility
- Maintain open communication with facility staff
- Participate in care planning meetings
- Monitor your loved one's care and speak up if you have concerns
- Continue to make decisions that align with your loved one's wishes

| Primary Caregiver Role | Advocate Role |
| --- | --- |
| Providing hands-on care | Ensuring quality of care |
| Managing daily routines | Participating in care planning |
| Administering medications | Monitoring medication management |
| Ensuring home safety | Assessing facility safety measures |

## Staying Involved After Facility Placement

**Your ongoing involvement is vital to your loved one's well-being in a care facility.** Here are ways to stay connected:

1. Visit regularly and at different times of day
2. Participate in facility activities with your loved one
3. Bring familiar items or photos to personalize their living space
4. Keep staff informed about your loved one's preferences and history
5. Maintain connections with other family members and friends
6. Celebrate holidays and special occasions together
7. Continue to advocate for your loved one's needs and preferences

Remember, your presence and involvement can significantly enhance your loved one's quality of life in a facility.

Deciding to move a loved one with dementia to a care facility is a profound act of love and commitment. It comes from wanting the best care and safety for your family member. As you navigate this challenging journey, be kind to yourself. Acknowledge the difficulty of the decision, but also recognize the courage it takes to make it.

Your role as a caregiver doesn't end with facility placement—it evolves. You'll continue to be vital to your loved one's care team, advocating for their needs and ensuring they receive the best possible care. This new chapter may bring challenges, but it can also give you peace of mind knowing your loved one receives professional care in a safe environment.

Remember, there's no "perfect" decision in this situation. The best decision is made with love, careful consideration, and a focus on your loved one's well-being. Trust in the process, lean on your support system and know you're doing your best for your loved one.

# Preparing for End-of-Life Decisions

While difficult to contemplate, preparing for end-of-life decisions is essential to caregiving. Having these conversations and making plans can provide peace of mind and ensure your loved one's wishes are respected.

**Steps in Preparing for End-of-Life Decisions:**

1. **Start the Conversation**
    - Choose a calm moment to discuss end-of-life wishes with your loved one.
    - Approach the topic with sensitivity and openness.

2. **Understand Your Loved One's Wishes**
    - Discuss preferences for medical interventions, pain management, and place of care.
    - Explore spiritual or cultural considerations.

3. **Document Decisions**
    - Ensure advance directives (living will, healthcare power of attorney) are in place.
    - Consider creating a POLST (Physician Orders for Life-Sustaining Treatment) form.

4. **Communicate with Healthcare Providers**
    - Share documented wishes with all relevant healthcare providers.
    - Ensure copies of advance directives are in medical records.

5. **Plan for Practical Matters**
    - Discuss funeral or memorial preferences.
    - Address financial and legal matters (wills, estate planning).

6. **Prepare Emotionally**
    - Seek support from counselors, support groups, or spiritual advisors.
    - Allow yourself to process emotions as you plan.
7. **Focus on Quality of Life**
    - Discuss what quality of life means to your loved one.
    - Align care decisions with these values.

| End-of-Life Consideration | Questions to Discuss | Documentation Needed |
|---|---|---|
| **Medical Interventions** | Preferences for resuscitation, ventilation, feeding tubes | Living Will, POLST Form |
| **Pain Management** | Comfort goals, medication preferences | Advance Directive, Pain Management Plan |
| **Place of Care** | Preference for home, hospital, or hospice care | Documented in Advance Care Plan |
| **Spiritual/Cultural Needs** | Desired rituals, religious support | Noted in Personal Directive |

Remember, coping with grief and loss is a profoundly personal journey. There's no right or wrong way to feel; seeking help is okay. By acknowledging your grief, finding meaning in your caregiving role, and preparing for difficult decisions, you're honoring both yourself and your loved one.

These conversations and preparations, while challenging, can bring a sense of peace and allow you to focus on creating meaningful moments with your loved one. Don't hesitate to lean on your support network, seek professional help if needed, and be gentle with yourself throughout this process. Your role as a caregiver is invaluable, and taking care of your emotional well-being is essential to providing compassionate care.

# When to Consider Hospice

**Hospice care** is a compassionate approach to end-of-life care that focuses on comfort, quality of life, and dignity. It's important to understand that choosing hospice doesn't mean giving up – it means shifting the focus from curative treatment to comfort care.

**Critical aspects of hospice care include:**

1. Pain management and symptom control
2. Emotional and spiritual support for the patient and family
3. Assistance with personal care and daily living activities
4. Respite care for family caregivers
5. Bereavement support for loved ones

**Hospice care is typically provided by a team of professionals, including:**

- Doctors
- Nurses
- Social workers
- Chaplains or spiritual advisors
- Trained volunteers

| Hospice Service | Description |
| --- | --- |
| **Medical Care** | Pain management, symptom control, and medication management. |
| **Personal Care** | Assistance with bathing, dressing, and other daily activities. |
| **Emotional Support** | Counseling for patient and family, addressing fears and concerns. |
| **Spiritual Care** | Support for spiritual needs and end-of-life rituals. |
| **Practical Support** | Help with household tasks, errands, and respite care. |

# The importance of timely hospice involvement

Deciding when to involve hospice care can be emotionally challenging, but **early involvement often leads to better outcomes** for both the person with dementia and their caregivers. Here's why timely hospice care is crucial:

1. **Improved quality of life**: Hospice teams are experts in managing pain and other symptoms, helping your loved one feel more comfortable.

2. **Reduced hospitalizations**: Proper symptom management often reduces the need for emergency room visits or hospital stays.

3. **Emotional and spiritual support**: Hospice offers counseling and support services that benefit you and your loved one.

4. **Time to say goodbye**: Earlier involvement gives family members more time to spend with their loved one and address unfinished business.

5. **Caregiver support**: Hospice provides education, resources, and respite care to help you navigate this challenging time.

Remember, choosing hospice doesn't mean death is imminent. Many patients receive hospice care for months, allowing them to make the most of their remaining time with improved comfort and quality of life.

| Benefits of Early Hospice Involvement | Impact on Patient and Family |
| --- | --- |
| **Better symptom management** | Increased comfort and reduced suffering |
| **Comprehensive support** | Improved overall quality of life for the patient and caregivers |
| **Avoid crises** | Less stress and anxiety for family members |
| **Time for meaningful moments** | Opportunity to create lasting memories and say goodbyes |

By understanding dementia, hospice care, and the benefits of timely involvement, you're better equipped to make informed decisions about your loved one's care. Remember, you're not alone in this journey – hospice teams are there to support both you and your loved one every step of the way.

# Signs It May Be Time for Hospice Care

As a caregiver or family member of someone with dementia, recognizing when it's time to consider hospice care can be challenging. This decision is deeply personal and often emotional. However, certain signs can help guide you in making this vital choice. Let's explore these indicators in detail.

## Physical indicators

Physical changes are often the most noticeable signs that your loved one's condition is progressing. **Look for these physical indicators**:

1. **Significant weight loss**: A 10% or more decrease in body weight in six months.

2. **Frequent infections**: Pneumonia or urinary tract infections that are becoming harder to treat.

3. **Difficulty swallowing**: This can lead to choking, coughing during meals, or refusal to eat.

4. **Increased pain**: Despite efforts to manage it with medication.

5. **Skin breakdown**: Pressure sores or other skin issues that aren't healing.

6. **Changes in breathing**: Shortness of breath, labored breathing, or long pauses between breaths.

7. **Decreased mobility**: Becoming bed-bound or unable to sit up without support.

| Physical Indicator | What to Look For |
| --- | --- |
| Weight Loss | Loose clothing, visible bone structure, sunken cheeks |
| Swallowing Difficulties | Coughing during meals, holding food in the mouth, refusing to eat |
| Skin Issues | Redness, open sores, slow healing of wounds |
| Mobility Changes | Inability to walk independently, frequent falls, reluctance to move |

## Cognitive and behavioral changes

As dementia progresses, you may notice significant changes in your loved one's cognitive abilities and behavior. **Fundamental changes to watch for include**:

- Increased confusion and disorientation
- Difficulty recognizing family members
- Loss of ability to communicate verbally
- Agitation, aggression, or combative behavior
- Withdrawal from social interactions
- Changes in sleep patterns (sleeping more during the day, restless at night)
- Hallucinations or delusions

Remember, these changes can be distressing for you and your loved one. Hospice care can help you manage these symptoms and improve your quality of life.

## Frequent hospitalizations or ER visits

If you find yourself taking your loved one to the emergency room or hospital more often, it might be time to consider hospice care. **Signs to consider include**:

1. Multiple hospitalizations within the past six months
2. Recurring infections or illnesses
3. Increasing difficulty managing symptoms at home
4. Longer recovery times after each hospital stay

| Frequency of Medical Visits | Consideration |
|---|---|
| **1-2 ER visits in 6 months** | Monitor closely and consult with a doctor. |
| **3+ ER visits in 6 months** | This is a strong indication for a hospice evaluation. |
| **Any hospital stay longer than one week** | Consider hospice discussion. |

## Decline in daily functioning

A significant decline in your loved one's ability to perform daily tasks independently is a strong indicator that hospice care may be beneficial. **Watch for**:

- Inability to dress, bathe, or groom without assistance
- Incontinence or loss of bladder and bowel control
- Difficulty moving from bed to chair without help
- Inability to prepare or eat meals independently
- Decreased interest in previously enjoyed activities

These changes often mean that your loved one requires more intensive care, which hospice can provide while ensuring comfort and dignity.

**In conclusion**, deciding when to consider hospice care is complex and personal. By being aware of these signs – physical changes, cognitive decline, frequent hospitalizations, and decreased daily functioning – you can make a more informed choice about when to seek additional support. Remember, hospice care is not about giving up hope; it's about ensuring the best possible quality of life for your loved one and support for you as a caregiver.

# The Benefits of Hospice Care for Dementia Patients

When considering hospice care for your loved one with dementia, it's essential to understand the numerous benefits this specialized care can provide. Hospice focuses on comfort and quality of life, offering a holistic approach to supporting the patient and their family. Let's explore these benefits in detail.

## Pain management and symptom control

One of the primary goals of hospice care is to ensure that your loved one is as comfortable as possible. **Effective pain management and symptom control can significantly improve their quality of life.**

Critical aspects of pain and symptom management in hospice care include:

1. **Personalized pain assessment**: Hospice professionals are trained to recognize pain in patients who cannot communicate verbally.

2. **Tailored medication plans**: Medications are carefully selected and adjusted to provide maximum comfort with minimal side effects.

3. **Non-pharmacological interventions** may include massage, music therapy, or aromatherapy to complement medication.

4. **Regular monitoring**: The hospice team assesses the patient's comfort level and adjusts care as needed.

5. **Management of other symptoms**: This includes addressing issues like shortness of breath, nausea, anxiety, and sleep disturbances.

| Common Dementia Symptoms | Hospice Management Approach |
|---|---|
| Pain | Tailored pain medication, positioning, gentle massage |
| Agitation | Calming techniques, environmental adjustments, medication if necessary |
| Difficulty swallowing | Dietary modifications, proper positioning, oral care |
| Skin issues | Regular repositioning, specialized mattresses, wound care |

### Emotional and spiritual support

Hospice care recognizes that emotional and spiritual well-being is as important as physical comfort. **This holistic approach can provide immense comfort to the patient and their family.**

Emotional and spiritual support in hospice care includes:

- Counseling services for the patient and family members
- Support from social workers to address practical and emotional concerns
- Chaplain services for spiritual support, regardless of religious affiliation
- Assistance with life review and legacy projects
- Grief counseling for family members, both before and after their loved one's passing

Remember, this support is tailored to your family's needs and beliefs. The hospice team is there to provide comfort and guidance, not to impose any particular spiritual or religious views.

## Respite care for family caregivers

Caring for a loved one with dementia can be physically and emotionally exhausting. **Hospice care recognizes the vital role of family caregivers and offers respite services to prevent burnout.**

Respite care benefits include:

1. Short-term relief from caregiving duties
2. Opportunity for self-care and rest
3. Time to attend to personal matters or other family responsibilities
4. Professional care for your loved one, ensuring their needs are met
5. Reduced stress and improved overall well-being for the caregiver

# Improved quality of life

The ultimate goal of hospice care is to improve the patient's and their family's overall quality of life. **This is achieved through expert care, support, and a focus on comfort rather than curative treatments.**

Ways hospice care can improve quality of life:

- Allowing the patient to remain in familiar surroundings, often at home
- Providing equipment and supplies necessary for comfort and care
- Offering 24/7 support and guidance for family caregivers
- Facilitating meaningful interactions and moments between the patient and their loved ones
- Ensuring dignity and respect in all aspects of care

| Addressing not just physical needs but also emotional, social, and spiritual needs Quality of Life Aspect | Hospice Care Impact |
|---|---|
| Comfort | Reduced pain and distressing symptoms. |
| Dignity | Personalized care respecting individual preferences. |
| Family connection | Support for meaningful interactions and memory-making. |
| Peace of mind | 24/7 professional support and guidance. |

In conclusion, hospice care offers numerous benefits for dementia patients and their families. By focusing on comprehensive symptom management, providing emotional and spiritual support, offering respite care, and striving to improve overall quality of life, hospice care can make a significant difference in your loved one's final months or years.

Remember, choosing hospice care doesn't mean giving up hope. Instead, it means shifting the focus to ensuring the best possible quality of life and comfort for your loved one. It's about making the most of your time together, creating meaningful moments, and finding peace in knowing your loved one receives expert, compassionate care.

# Common Misconceptions About Hospice Care

When considering hospice care for a loved one with dementia, you may encounter several misconceptions that can cause hesitation or concern. Understanding the realities of hospice care is essential to making an informed decision. Let's address the most common misconceptions and clarify what hospice care entails.

## Hospice is not giving up.

One of the most pervasive misconceptions about hospice care is that it means "giving up" on your loved one. **This couldn't be further from the truth.**

Here's why hospice is not giving up:

1. **Shift in focus**: Hospice represents a change in care goals, not an abandonment of care. The focus shifts from curative treatments to comfort and quality of life.

2. **Active care**: Hospice provides expert care to manage symptoms and improve comfort.

3. **A holistic approach** addresses not just physical needs but also emotional, social, and spiritual aspects of well-being.

4. **Empowerment**: Hospice empowers patients and families to make choices about their care and how they want to spend their remaining time.

5. **Celebration of life**: Many hospice programs encourage life reviews and legacy projects, which celebrate the person's life and accomplishments.

| Misconception | Reality |
| --- | --- |
| **Hospice means no more treatment.** | Hospice provides active treatment for symptoms and comfort. |
| **Choosing hospice means giving up hope.** | Hospice shifts hope to quality of life and meaningful moments. |
| **Hospice is only for the last few days of life.** | Hospice can provide care for months, enhancing life quality. |

## Hospice doesn't mean imminent death.

Another common misconception is that hospice care is only for the last few days or weeks of life. **Hospice care can be beneficial for months and sometimes even longer.**

Key points to understand:

- Hospice eligibility typically requires a prognosis of six months or less, but this is not a strict limit.
- Many patients receive hospice care for several months, with some even "graduating" from hospice if their condition stabilizes.
- Earlier involvement of hospice often leads to a better quality of life and can sometimes even extend life by reducing stress on the body.
- Hospice care can be discontinued if the patient's condition improves or if they decide to pursue curative treatments again.

| Time in Hospice | Potential Benefits |
| --- | --- |
| **Days to weeks** | Immediate comfort care and family support in crisis |
| **Weeks to months** | Sustained symptom management, quality time with family |
| **Months or longer** | Long-term comfort, potential for stabilization or improvement |

## Hospice care can be provided at home.

Many people believe that choosing hospice care means their loved one must move to a facility. **Hospice care is often provided right in the comfort of the patient's home.**

Understanding home hospice care:

1. **Flexibility**: Hospice care can be provided wherever the patient calls home – private residences, assisted living facilities, or nursing homes.
2. **Customized care**: The hospice team works with you to create a care plan that fits your home environment and family dynamics.
3. **Equipment and supplies**: Necessary medical equipment (like hospital beds or oxygen) is provided and set up in the home.

4. **24/7 support**: While the hospice team isn't present 24/7, they're always available by phone for guidance and can visit as needed.

5. **Family involvement**: Home hospice allows family members to be intimately involved in care, with guidance from the hospice team.

6. **Familiar surroundings**: Patients often find comfort surrounded by familiar sights, sounds, and loved ones.

| Aspect of Care | In-Home Hospice Provision |
| --- | --- |
| **Medical care** | Regular visits from nurses and doctors |
| **Personal care** | Assistance with bathing and dressing by hospice aides |
| **Emotional support** | Visits from social workers and counselors |
| **Spiritual care** | Chaplain visits if desired |

It's important to note that while home hospice is common, inpatient hospice facilities are available for those who need or prefer that option. Some patients may transition between home and inpatient care as their needs change.

In conclusion, understanding these common misconceptions about hospice care can help you make a more informed decision for your loved one with dementia. Hospice is not about giving up or waiting for death; it's about living life as fully and comfortably as possible in whatever time remains. It offers expert care that can often be provided at home, surrounding your loved one with familiar comforts and loving family members.

Remember, choosing hospice care is a profoundly personal decision. It's okay to have questions and concerns. Don't hesitate to contact hospice providers in your area to learn more about their services and how they might benefit your loved one and your family. Your choice to consider hospice care demonstrates your commitment to ensuring the best possible quality of life for your loved one, which is an act of profound love and care.

# How to Initiate the Hospice Conversation

Initiating a conversation about hospice care can be challenging and emotionally charged. However, having these discussions early can lead to better care decisions and more time to prepare. Here's how to approach this sensitive topic with compassion and clarity.

## Talking with your loved one

When possible, it's essential to involve your loved one with dementia in the decision-making process. While their ability to participate may vary, including them shows respect for their wishes and autonomy.

## Tips for talking with your loved one:

1. **Choose the right time and place**: Find a quiet, comfortable setting where your loved one is most alert and receptive.

2. **Be direct but gentle**: Use clear, simple language. Avoid euphemisms that might confuse them.

3. **Listen actively**: Pay attention to their verbal and non-verbal responses.

4. **Respect their feelings**: Acknowledge any fears or concerns they express.

5. **Focus on the benefits**: Explain how hospice can help manage their symptoms and improve comfort.

6. **Be patient.** This may need to be an ongoing conversation. Don't rush to decide everything in one sitting.

**Use visual aids:** If appropriate, consider using brochures or videos to help explain hospice care.

**What to Say** / **What to Avoid**

| What to Say | What to Avoid |
|---|---|
| "I want to talk about how we can keep you comfortable." | "We need to discuss end-of-life care." |
| "Hospice can help us manage your pain better." | "There's nothing more we can do for you." |
| "What's most important to you right now?" | "You should consider hospice care." |

## Discussing with family members

Bringing up hospice care with other family members can sometimes be as challenging as discussing it with your loved one. Family dynamics, differing opinions, and emotional responses can complicate these conversations.

**Strategies for family discussions:**

- **Plan**: Consider who should be part of the conversation and how to involve distant family members.

- **Choose a spokesperson**: Designate one person to lead the conversation if helpful.

- **Share information**: Before the discussion, provide educational materials about hospice care to all family members.

- **Be inclusive**: Ensure everyone has a chance to express their thoughts and feelings.

- **Focus on your loved one's wishes**: If known, center the discussion on what your loved one with dementia would want.

- **Address concerns**: Be open to questions and address fears or misconceptions about hospice care.

**Seek professional help:** Consider involving a social worker or counselor to facilitate the conversation if family conflicts arise.

**Common Family Concerns** | **Possible Responses**

| | |
|---|---|
| "Isn't this giving up?" | "Hospice focuses on quality of life and comfort, not giving up." |
| "It's too soon to consider hospice." | "Earlier hospice involvement often leads to better care and support." |
| "We can't afford it." | "Medicare, Medicaid, and most private insurances usually cover hospice." |

## Consulting with healthcare providers

Healthcare providers play a crucial role in the decision to pursue hospice care. They can provide valuable insights into your loved one's condition and prognosis and help you understand if hospice is appropriate.

**Steps for consulting healthcare providers:**

1. **Schedule a dedicated appointment**: Request a meeting to discuss your loved one's care options, including hospice.

2. **Prepare questions**: Write down your questions and concerns beforehand. Some key questions might include:
   - Is my loved one eligible for hospice care?
   - How might hospice benefit them at this stage?
   - What changes in their condition should we be watching for?

3. **Bring support**: Consider having another family member present to help remember information.

4. **Take notes**: Write down important points or ask if you can record the conversation for future reference.

5. **Discuss prognosis**: While difficult, understanding the expected progression of your loved one's condition can help you make decisions.

6. **Ask about referrals**: If hospice seems appropriate, ask for referrals to reputable hospice providers in your area.

7. **Follow-up**: Don't hesitate to contact the healthcare provider with any additional questions after the meeting.

| Healthcare Provider | Role in Hospice Discussion |
| --- | --- |
| Primary Care Physician | Overall health assessment and long-term care planning. |
| Neurologist | Dementia progression and symptom management. |
| Geriatrician | Specialized care needs for older adults. |
| Palliative Care Specialist | Expert in comfort care and quality of life issues. |

Remember, initiating the hospice conversation is an act of love and care. It shows that you're thinking proactively about ensuring the best possible quality of life for your loved one. While these discussions can be difficult, they often bring a sense of relief and clarity once they're underway.

It's normal to feel a range of emotions during this process. Don't hesitate to seek support for yourself, whether from friends, support groups, or professional counselors. Taking care of your emotional well-being is crucial as you navigate this challenging journey.

Ultimately, the goal is to make informed decisions that honor your loved one's wishes and provide them with the most appropriate and compassionate care possible. By approaching these conversations with openness, empathy, and a focus on your loved one's well-being, you can navigate this critical decision-making process with greater confidence and peace of mind.

# The Hospice Evaluation Process

Understanding the hospice evaluation process can help alleviate some of the anxiety and uncertainty you may feel when considering this option for your loved one with dementia. This process ensures that hospice care is appropriate and tailored to your loved one's specific needs. Let's explore each step in detail.

## Eligibility criteria for dementia patients

Specific criteria apply to people with dementia who are eligible for hospice care. **These criteria are guidelines, and each case is evaluated individually.**

Key eligibility factors for dementia patients include:

1. **Disease progression**: The person should be in the late stages of dementia, typically stage 7, on the Functional Assessment Staging Test (FAST).

2. **Functional decline**: Inability to perform daily activities without substantial assistance.

3. **Medical complications**: Presence of conditions such as aspiration pneumonia, upper urinary tract infections, sepsis, or multiple stage 3-4 pressure ulcers.

4. **Nutritional decline**: Difficulty eating and swallowing, leading to weight loss.

5. **Verbal communication**: Limited to fewer than six intelligible daily words.

6. **Mobility**: Unable to walk without assistance and eventually becoming bed-bound.

| Eligibility Factor | Description |
|---|---|
| FAST Stage 7 | Very severe cognitive decline, minimal verbal communication |
| ADL Dependence | Requires help with most or all activities of daily living |
| Medical Complications | Recurrent infections, difficulty swallowing, pressure sores |
| Nutritional Decline | Significant weight loss, difficulty eating independently |

Remember, meeting these criteria doesn't automatically mean hospice is the right choice, nor does failing to meet all requirements necessarily disqualify someone. The decision involves a comprehensive evaluation by healthcare professionals and discussions with the family.

## What to expect during the evaluation

The hospice evaluation is a thorough process designed to assess your loved one's needs and determine whether hospice care is appropriate. **It is typically provided at no cost and does not obligate you to choose hospice care.**

The evaluation process usually includes:

- **Initial consultation**: A hospice representative will meet with you and your loved one to explain services and answer questions.

- **Medical review**: The hospice team will review your loved one's medical history and condition.

- **Physical assessment**: A nurse will conduct a physical examination to evaluate symptoms and care needs.

- **Psychosocial assessment**: A social worker may assess emotional needs and family dynamics.

- **Home safety evaluation**: If care will be provided at home, the team will assess the environment for safety and equipment needs.

- **Discussion of goals**: The team will discuss your loved one's care goals and preferences with you.

| Evaluation Step | Conducted By |
|---|---|
| **Initial Consultation** | Hospice Representative |
| **Medical Review** | Hospice Physician |
| **Physical Assessment** | Hospice Nurse |
| **Psychosocial Assessment** | Social Worker |

# Creating a care plan

If your loved one is found eligible for hospice and you decide to proceed, the next step is creating a personalized care plan. This plan is a **collaborative effort** between the hospice team, your loved one (if able to participate), and your family.

The care plan typically includes:

1. **Symptom management strategies**: Plans for managing pain, anxiety, breathing difficulties, and other symptoms.
2. **Medication regimen**: A review and adjustment of current medications, focusing on comfort and symptom control.
3. **Personal care routines**: Plans for bathing, feeding, and other daily care needs.
4. **Emotional and spiritual support**: Arrange counseling, chaplain visits, or other support services.
5. **Family education**: Training for family caregivers on providing care and recognizing important signs or symptoms.
6. **Emergency procedures**: Clear instructions on what to do in case of emergencies or sudden changes in condition.
7. **Respite care arrangements**: Plans for providing breaks to family caregivers.

| Care Plan Component | Purpose |
| --- | --- |
| Symptom Management | Ensure comfort and quality of life. |
| Medication Management | Optimize effectiveness and minimize side effects. |
| Personal Care | Maintain dignity and prevent complications. |
| Emotional Support | Address the psychological needs of the patient and family. |

It's important to understand that the care plan is a **dynamic document**. It will be regularly reviewed and adjusted as your loved one's needs change. You and your family will be integral parts of this ongoing process.

Remember, the hospice evaluation and care planning process ensures your loved one receives the most appropriate and compassionate care possible. It's an opportunity to ask questions, express concerns, and actively participate in shaping your loved one's care.

Don't hesitate to ask for clarification if anything is unclear during this process. The hospice team supports you and your loved one every step of the way. They aim to honor your loved one's wishes, provide expert care, and help your entire family through this challenging time.

By understanding and actively participating in the evaluation and care planning process, you're taking an essential step in ensuring the best possible care and quality of life for your loved one with dementia. While sometimes emotional, this process can also bring relief and clarity as you navigate this difficult journey.

# Preparing for Hospice Care

Once you've decided to pursue hospice care for your loved one with dementia, there are several important steps to take to ensure a smooth transition. This preparation phase is crucial for creating a supportive environment and understanding what to expect. Let's explore these steps in detail.

## Choosing a Hospice Provider

Selecting the right hospice provider is a critical decision that can significantly impact the quality of care your loved one receives. **Take your time with this process, and don't hesitate to ask questions.**

Consider the following when choosing a hospice provider:

1. **Certification and accreditation**: Ensure the provider is Medicare-certified and, ideally, accredited by a national organization.

2. **Range of services**: Look for providers offering comprehensive medical, emotional, and spiritual support.

3. **Availability**: Choose a provider that offers 24/7 emergency on-call services.

4. **Experience with dementia**: Ask about their specific experience in caring for patients with dementia.

5. **Staff qualifications**: Inquire about the training and qualifications of their care team members.

6. **Respite care options**: Check if they offer respite care to give family caregivers breaks.

7. **Bereavement support**: Look for providers that offer grief counseling and support after your loved one's passing.

| Question to Ask | Why It's Important |
| --- | --- |
| How quickly can you start services? | Ensures timely care initiation |
| What is your staff-to-patient ratio? | Indicates the level of individual attention |
| How do you manage pain in dementia patients? | Reveals expertise in dementia-specific care |
| What support do you offer family caregivers? | Indicates the level of family involvement and support |

## Setting up the care environment

Creating a safe, comfortable environment is essential for hospice care, especially if your loved one will be cared for at home. **The goal is to promote comfort, safety, and ease of care.**

Critical considerations for setting up the care environment:

- **Bedroom setup**: Ensure the bed is accessible from both sides. If recommended by the hospice team, consider a hospital bed.

- **Bathroom modifications**: Install grab bars, a raised toilet seat, and non-slip mats if needed.

- **Clear pathways**: Remove clutter and ensure clear paths for easy movement, primarily if a wheelchair or walker is used.

- **Lighting**: Provide adequate lighting to prevent falls and aid in care tasks.

- **Comfortable seating**: Have a comfortable chair for your loved one and seating for visitors.

- **Temperature control**: Ensure the room can be kept at a comfortable temperature.

- **Meaningful objects**: Include photos, favorite blankets, or other cherished items to create a comforting atmosphere.

| Item | Purpose |
| --- | --- |
| **Hospital bed** | Allows for positioning adjustments, easier care |
| **Bedside commode** | Reduces the need for bathroom trips |
| **Over-bed table** | Provides surface for meals, activities |
| **Night light** | Improves safety during nighttime care |

## Understanding your role as a caregiver

As a family caregiver, your role will evolve with the introduction of hospice care. **While the hospice team will provide expert care, your involvement remains crucial.**

Your role as a caregiver may include:

1. **Being an advocate**: You know your loved one best. Share insights about their preferences, behaviors, and needs with the hospice team.

2. **Providing comfort**: Your presence and touch can be incredibly comforting. Spend time with your loved one, hold their hand, or sit with them.

3. **Assisting with personal care**: The hospice team will guide you in helping with feeding, bathing, or repositioning.

4. **Medication management**: While the hospice team will manage medications, you may be involved in administering them.

5. **Emotional support**: Provide reassurance and emotional support to your loved one.

6. **Communication liaison**: Keep other family members informed about your loved one's condition and care.

7. **Self-care**: Remember to take care of yourself too. Accept help and take breaks when needed.

| Caregiver Task | Hospice Team Support |
| --- | --- |
| **Personal care assistance** | Training on safe techniques, along with regular help from hospice aides |
| **Medication administration** | Clear instructions, regular check-ins, 24/7 phone support |
| **Emotional support** | Counseling services, tips for communication |
| **Recognizing changes in condition** | Education on what to watch for, when to call for help |

Remember, the hospice team supports you and your loved one. **Don't hesitate to ask for help or clarification when you need it.** They can provide training, answer questions, and support you as you navigate this new role.

Preparing for hospice care can feel overwhelming, but taking these steps can help create a smoother transition. By choosing the right provider, setting up a comfortable environment, and understanding your role, you're laying the groundwork for compassionate, quality care for your loved one.

This preparation phase is also a time for emotional readiness. It's normal to feel a mix of emotions – relief, sadness, anxiety, or even guilt. Remember that choosing hospice care is an act of love, focusing on comfort and quality of life for your loved one. Don't hesitate to lean on the hospice team, friends, or support groups for emotional support.

By taking these steps to prepare, you're ensuring that your loved one will receive the best possible care in their final stage of life while also setting yourself up to be an informed and supported caregiver. Your dedication to this process is a testament to your love and commitment to your family member's well-being.

# Navigating the Emotional Journey

The decision to pursue hospice care for a loved one with dementia marks the beginning of a profound emotional journey. This period can be filled with complex feelings and challenges. Understanding these emotions and finding coping methods is crucial for you and your loved one. Let's explore this journey and discuss strategies for navigating it with resilience and grace.

## Coping with grief and anticipatory loss

Grief is a natural response to loss, and it often begins well before the actual passing of a loved one. This is known as anticipatory grief. **Recognizing and acknowledging these feelings is an essential step in coping with them.**

Common experiences of anticipatory grief include:

- Sadness and tearfulness
- Anxiety about the future
- Anger or frustration
- Guilt over past events or current feelings
- A sense of helplessness
- Difficulty concentrating
- Physical symptoms like fatigue or changes in appetite

Strategies for coping with anticipatory grief:

1. **Acknowledge your feelings**: Allow yourself to feel whatever emotions arise without judgment.
2. **Share your feelings**: Talk to trusted friends, family members, or a professional counselor.
3. **Practice self-compassion**: Be kind to yourself. Grief is a normal and valid response to your situation.
4. **Stay connected**: Maintain relationships with friends and family. Don't isolate yourself.
5. **Take care of your physical health**: Eat well, exercise, and get enough sleep.
6. **Find healthy outlets**: Engage in activities that help you process your emotions, such as journaling, art, or music.

7. **Stay present**: While worrying about the future is natural, focus on the present moment and your time with your loved one.

| Grief Response | Coping Strategy |
|---|---|
| Overwhelming sadness | Allow yourself to cry; talk to a supportive friend. |
| Anxiety about the future | Practice mindfulness; focus on one day at a time. |
| Guilt over negative feelings | Practice self-compassion; join a support group. |
| Physical exhaustion | Prioritize self-care; ask for help with tasks. |

## Finding support for caregivers

Caring for a loved one with dementia in hospice care can be emotionally and physically demanding. **Seeking support is not a sign of weakness but a necessary step in maintaining your well-being.**

Options for caregiver support include:

- **Support groups**: Join groups specifically for dementia caregivers or hospice families. These can be in-person or online.
- **Professional counseling**: Consider individual therapy to process emotions and develop coping strategies.
- **Respite care**: Take your hospice provider's respite services for necessary breaks.
- **Family and friends**: Don't hesitate to ask for and accept help from your support network.
- **Educational resources**: Attend workshops or webinars about caregiving and end-of-life care to feel more prepared.
- **Spiritual or religious support**: If applicable, seek guidance from spiritual leaders or faith communities.
- **Self-care activities**: Engage in activities that recharge you, even for short periods.

| Type of Support | Benefits |
| --- | --- |
| Caregiver support groups | Shared experiences, practical tips, emotional validation. |
| Professional counseling | Personalized coping strategies and safe space to process emotions. |
| Respite care | Time for self-care and reduced burnout risk. |
| Educational resources | Increased confidence in caregiving, better preparedness. |

## Celebrating life and creating meaningful moments

While this time is undoubtedly challenging, it also presents opportunities to celebrate your loved one's life and create lasting memories. **Focusing on positive experiences can provide comfort and meaning during this challenging journey.**

Ideas for creating meaningful moments:

1. **Life review**: Remember happy memories, perhaps creating a scrapbook or memory box together.

2. **Music therapy**: Play your loved one's favorite songs or hymns. Music can often evoke positive responses, even in late-stage dementia.

3. **Sensory experiences**: Engage the senses with familiar scents, textures, or flavors that bring comfort.

4. **Nature connection**: If possible, spend time outdoors or bring nature inside with flowers or plants.

5. **Gentle touch**: Hold hands, give a soft massage, or sit close to provide comfort through touch.

6. **Family gatherings**: Organize small, quiet gatherings of close family and friends to share stories and love.

7. **Legacy projects**: Create something together that can be shared with future generations, like a recipe book or family tree.

8. **Spiritual practices**: If prayer, meditation, or other spiritual practices are essential to your loved one, engage in them.

| Meaningful Activity | Potential Benefits |
| --- | --- |
| Looking at old photos | Stimulates memories and encourages storytelling. |
| Listening to favorite music | It evokes emotions and may improve mood. |
| Gentle hand massage | It provides comfort and promotes relaxation. |
| Reading aloud familiar stories | Offers comfort and maintains connection. |

Remember, the goal is not to create grand gestures but to find moments of connection, comfort, and joy, however small they seem.

Navigating the emotional journey of hospice care for a loved one with dementia is undoubtedly challenging. It's a path filled with complex emotions, difficult decisions, and profound moments of love and connection. You can find strength and moments of peace by acknowledging your feelings, seeking support, and focusing on creating meaningful experiences.

It's important to remember that there's no "right" way to feel or grieve. Your journey is unique, and having good and bad days is okay. Be patient and compassionate with yourself as you navigate this path.

Lastly, don't forget that the hospice team supports you and your loved one. They can provide resources, counseling, and guidance to help you through this emotional journey. You're not alone in this process; reaching out for help when needed is a sign of strength and love for yourself and your loved one.

# Legal and Financial Considerations

When caring for a loved one with dementia who is entering hospice care, it's important to consider legal and financial matters. These can be challenging topics, but planning can bring peace of mind and help avoid problems later. Let's look at some key things to consider.

## Advance Directives and Power of Attorney

Advance directives say what kind of medical care your loved one wants if they can't speak for themselves. There are two main types:

1. Living Will: This document states what medical treatments your loved one wants or doesn't want at the end of life.
2. Healthcare Power of Attorney: This names someone to make medical decisions if your loved one can't.

Power of attorney is also crucial for money matters. It lets someone manage your loved one's finances if they can't do it themselves.

Why these papers matter:

- They make sure your loved one's wishes are followed
- They can prevent family arguments about care decisions
- They make it easier to handle bills and other money matters

Setting these up early is best while your loved one can still make decisions. If you haven't done this yet, talk to a lawyer who knows about elder law as soon as possible.

| Document | What It Does |
| --- | --- |
| **Living Will** | States end-of-life care wishes |
| **Healthcare Power of Attorney** | Names someone to make medical decisions |
| **Financial Power of Attorney** | Names someone to handle money matters |

## Understanding Hospice Coverage and Costs

The good news is that Medicare, Medicaid, and most private insurance plans usually cover hospice care. This coverage includes:

- Doctor and nursing services
- Medical equipment and supplies
- Medications for symptom control and pain relief
- Short-term inpatient care, if needed
- Grief counseling for the patient and family

What's not covered:

- Room and board if the patient is at home or in a nursing facility
- Treatments aimed at curing the illness (instead of comfort care); such treatments can invalidate hospice services.

It's good to check with your hospice provider and insurance company to understand what's covered and what you might need to pay for.

| Usually Covered | Usually Not Covered |
|---|---|
| **Hospice team visits** | Curative treatments (which can invalidate hospice services) |
| **Medical equipment** | Room and board at home |
| **Medications for comfort** | Care from providers outside the hospice |

## Additional Resources and Support Programs

Besides insurance, other programs might help with costs or provide extra support:

1. Veterans Benefits: If your loved one served in the military, they might qualify for special hospice benefits through the VA.

2. Social Security: Your loved one might be eligible for disability benefits if they're under 65.

3. Local Senior Services: Many communities have programs that offer seniors meals, transportation, or other help.

4. Alzheimer's Association: They offer support groups and education and can help you find local resources.

5. Area Agency on Aging: This government program can connect you with services in your area.

Don't be afraid to ask for help. Social workers at the hospice or your local senior center can often recommend programs that might help.

| Resource | What It Offers |
| --- | --- |
| **Veterans Benefits** | Special hospice care for veterans |
| **Social Security** | Possible disability benefits |
| **Alzheimer's Association** | Support groups and education |

Remember, dealing with legal and money matters can feel overwhelming, but it's integral to caring for your loved one. Don't hesitate to ask for help from professionals like lawyers, financial advisors, or social workers. They can guide you through these complex issues and help you make the best decisions for your family.

# Conclusion

As you reach the end of ***Placement for Dementia: A Dementia Care Essentials Guide***, take a moment to acknowledge the profound journey you are on as a caregiver. Navigating the complexities of dementia care is a testament to your strength, compassion, and dedication. This book provides the tools and insights to make informed decisions about facility placement, ensuring the best care for your loved one.

Remember, the challenges you face are not a reflection of your abilities but a testament to the depth of your commitment. It's natural to experience various emotions, from stress to uncertainty. Embrace these feelings with self-compassion and recognize the importance of caring for yourself. Your well-being is crucial not only for your health but also for the quality of care you provide.

As you continue this journey, seek support from fellow caregivers, utilize respite services, and prioritize self-care. Remember, asking for help is a sign of strength, not weakness. By nurturing your health, you enhance your capacity to offer the love, patience, and support your loved one deserves.

In closing, your role as a caregiver is invaluable. Thank you for your unwavering dedication and the kindness you bring to this challenging yet rewarding journey. With the knowledge and strategies gained from this guide, may you find clarity, comfort, and confidence in your decisions for your loved one.

# Resources

## Associations

Alzheimer's Association at https://www.alz.org/

Dementia Society of America at http://www.dementiasociety.org

National Institute on Aging at https://www.nia.nih.gov/

National Alliance for Caregiving at http://www.caregiving.org

Family Caregiver Alliance at http://www.caregiver.org

American Sleep Apnea Association at https://www.sleepapnea.org/

# Author Bio

 Peter Abraham, BSN, RN is an experienced nurse dedicated to supporting nurses, caregivers, families, and patients in their learning, growth, and well-being journey. Peter's nursing path encompasses practical experience as a cardiac telemetry nurse in a bustling cardiology unit at a Magnet-awarded teaching hospital. Additionally, Peter has fulfilled the role of a second-shift RN supervisor, overseeing an entire building in an SNF/LTC (Skilled Nursing Facility/Long-Term Care) setting with 151 residents. Remarkably, during the initial wave of COVID-19, the facility achieved an impressive close-to-100% recovery rate before operation warp speed was complete.

Furthermore, Peter's nursing career extends to rural home hospice care. As a visiting hospice registered nurse case manager, he offers compassionate care to patients in various settings, including private homes, personal care homes, assisted living facilities, skilled nursing facilities, and hospitals.

Moreover, Peter's desire to help others extends beyond his physical presence. At CompassionCrossing.Info, he writes articles to empower caregivers, family members, and fellow nurses in end-of-life care. Peter's drive to help others, which flows from his love of Christ Jesus, is a source of support and encouragement for all he reaches.

Other books by Peter Abraham include the following:

**Empowering Excellence in Hospice: A Nurse's Toolkit for Best Practices** series:

> Compliance-based, Eligibility Driven Hospice Documentation: Tips for Hospice Nurses
> Whispers of Time: Understanding the End-of-Life Timeline
> Terminal Clarity: Hospice Eligibility Guide for Nurses

**Compassionate Caregiving** series:

> Daily Hospice Care Planner: Organize, Communicate, and Provide Consistent Care
> Dignity in Dying: A Thoughtful Approach to Voluntary Stopping Eating and Drinking
> Palliative Sedation: A Compassionate Approach
> Hospice Medication Handbook: A Caregiver's Guide to Comfort Medications

**Dementia Caregivers Essentials** series:

> CPAP and Oxygen for Dementia
> Diabetes Care for Dementia
> Hallucination Management for Dementia
> Medication Compliance for Dementia
> Nutrition for Dementia
> Placement for Dementia
> Sundowning Management for Dementia

Connect with Peter On:

Website: https://compassioncrossing.info/

www.ingramcontent.com/pod-product-compliance
Lightning Source LLC
Chambersburg PA
CBHW050259230526
45471CB00005B/1959